11.41

CONTROL YOUR
ACIDITY
THE ACID/BASE DIET

**Correct your food in order to purify your body
and prevent from deceases**

D1373015

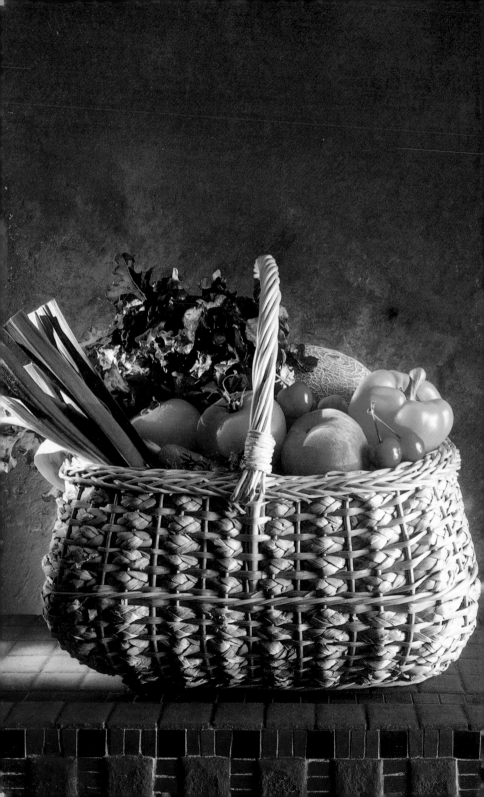

CONTROL YOUR
ACIDITY
THE ACID/BASE DIET

**Correct your food in order to purify your body
and prevent from deceases**

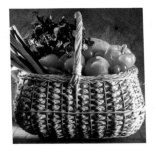

Dr Max Rombi

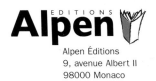

Alpen Éditions
9, avenue Albert II
98000 Monaco

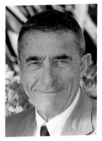

Dr Max Rombi is the creator of the Virbac Veterinary Company and of the Laboratoires Arkopharma, which have since become world leaders in phytotherapy and alternative medicine. Arkocaps have enjoyed a success that has spread worldwide. Dr Rombi believes that people must always be informed so that they can take their own health in hand.

From the same author:
the XXL Syndrome, Alpen Éditions.

Exclusive copyrights:
© Alpen Éditions
9, avenue Albert II
MC - 98000 MONACO
Tel: 00377 97 77 62 10
Fax: 00377 97 77 62 11
Web: www.alpen.mc

Managing Publisher: Christophe Didierlaurent
Editorial: Fabienne Desmarets and Sandra Del Barba
Designer: Stéphane Falaschi

Copyrights:
Banana Stock, Brand X, BSIP, Corbis, Goodshoot,
Image source, Stockbyte, Think Stock, Photo Alto, Photodisc
Artwork: © Sébastien Telleschi

ISBN13: 978-2-35934-064-8

JUN ¿ 4 2011

Printed in Italy

Introduction

The concept of acidity or alkalinity is difficult to understand without a bit of chemistry.

You are certainly familiar with the sour taste of lemons, but on the other hand, you are probably unfamiliar with the taste of acidic or alkaline products.

All of this boils down to chemistry. You should know that water, which makes up 60% of your body and circulates throughout it in the form of blood and lymph, has the chemical formula H_2O (H-O-H). Therefore, this molecule is made up of two parts: $H+$ and $OH-$.

If you dissolve sulfuric acid, SO_4H_2, in water, it splits into SO_4- and $2H+$.

If you dissolve caustic potash (KOH) in water, it splits into $K+$ and $OH-$.

The more $H+$ ions there are in a solution, the more acidic the solution is (see page on measuring pH). The other way around, if a solution is rich in $OH-$ ions, the more alkaline (or basic) it is.

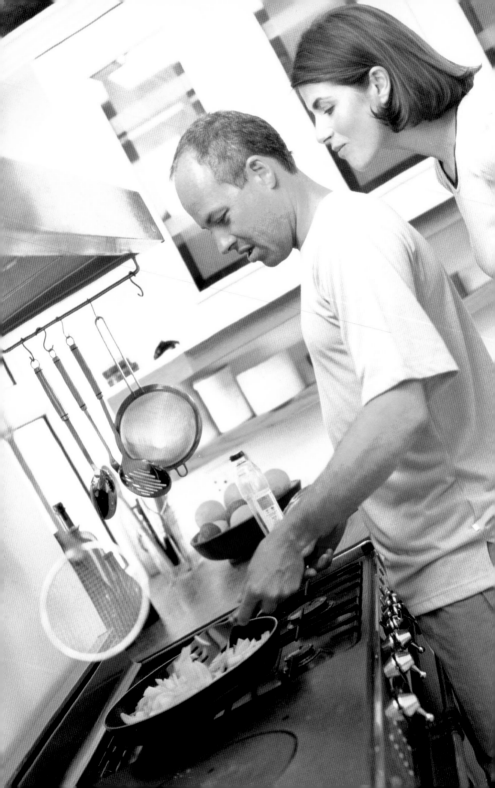

The mystery of acid-base balance has now been solved : it is a battle between H+ and OH-. We are going to attempt to explain all of this to you.

TABLE OF CONTENTS

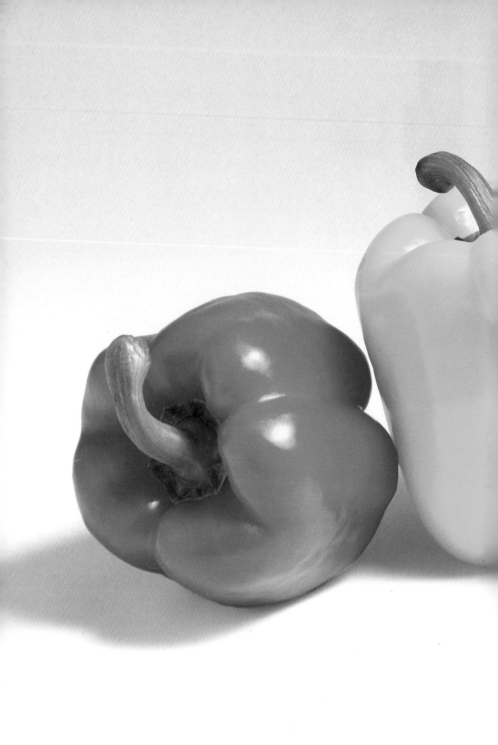

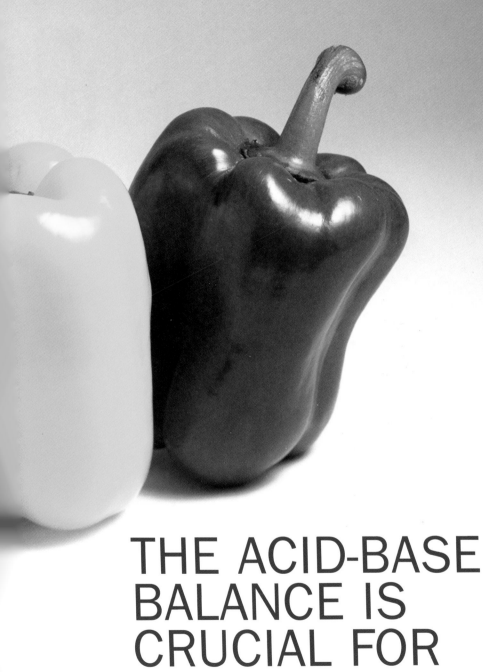

THE ACID-BASE
BALANCE IS
CRUCIAL FOR
YOUR HEALTH

Why do we speak of an acid-base balance?

To survive and function effectively, your body's cells require a relatively constant temperature, pressure, and also... acidity.

In order for human beings to survive, the physical and chemical conditions of their internal environment must be maintained relatively constant. Our blood volume should be constant, our body temperature must remain at 98.6°F (37°C), and our blood pressure should be approximately 120/80mmHg. The same goes for another parameter, which is the **acidity** of our body fluids. Our body has the ability to maintain a constant acidity both inside and outside its cells. This is known as the **acid-base balance.**.

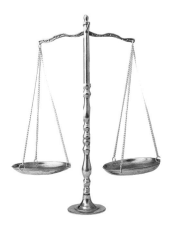

A vital balance

The acid-base balance is extremely important for your health, as it is essential for the normal functioning of each and every one of your cells. Indeed, the chemical reactions that are necessary for life, also known as enzymatic reactions, are generally sensitive to the acidity of the environment in which they occur. If you take into account that each cell contains thousands of different enzymes, each of which is in charge of a specific reaction, it is easy to understand how important this balance really is.

A number of important biological functions such as digestion, respiration, and cellular metabolism also depend on this balance.

Several body systems contribute to maintaining this balance: the kidneys, lungs, and digestive tract. If these systems function correctly – your body compensates for each time you consume acidifying substances so as to maintain the balance. If this happens, your cells can survive and function efficiently. However, if the systems' functioning is disturbed, the internal environment's makeup may change, and the balance is offset. This is the beginning of a vicious cycle.

This guide is aimed at demonstrating how the cells are unable to function efficiently when this acid-base balance is disturbed. Should this occur, the cells lose their vitality, and vital processes are jeopardized. In the long term, this imbalance can lead to chronic diseases.

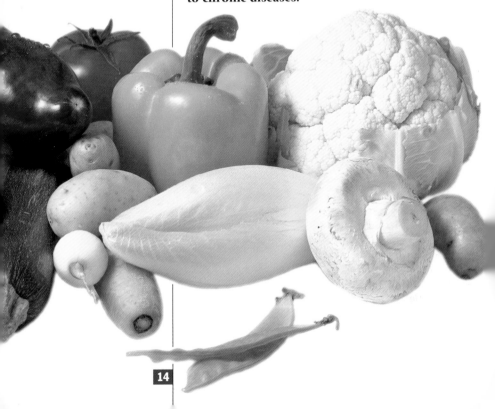

Where do acidifying substances come from ?

They are found in what we eat. Our diet's role is providing our body with the energy it needs, but changing food into energy is not where the process ends. This process creates waste, some of which is acidic. The acid burden that our body deals with every day depends on the quality of our diet, and to some extent, on our lifestyle. In order to neutralize this excess acid efficiently, we need to eat a balanced diet. Our diet and lifestyle are at the very center of our acid-base balance.

Fluids in the body

Water makes up about 60% of our body weight. It is classified into intracellular (the water found within the cells, about 40% of our body weight), and extracellular liquid (20% of our body weight), which surrounds the cells, notably the blood and lymph.
There is a balance between these two liquid components, which differ with respect to their composition and acidity.

Acids, bases, and pH

We have all heard about acids, bases, and pH, but what do these terms really mean and why are they important ?

An **acid** is a substance which releases hydrogen ions (H+)
A **base** is a substance which accepts hydrogen ions.
The concentration of hydrogen ions in a solution determines its acidity. Acidity is measured on a scale, which is known as the pH scale. This scale ranges from 0 to 14. As the concentration of hydrogen ions increases, the pH value decreases.
The more acidic the solution, the lower the pH value. Similarly, pH values higher than 7 correspond to alkaline solutions (less acid); the higher the pH value, the more alkaline (basic) the solution

Fig. 1 – pH scale

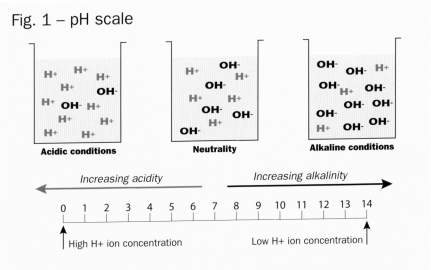

Acidic conditions Neutrality Alkaline conditions

Increasing acidity Increasing alkalinity

0 1 2 3 4 5 6 7 8 9 10 11 12 13 14

High H+ ion concentration Low H+ ion concentration

Values lower than 7 are indicative of an acid solution, and values higher than 7 are indicative of an alkaline (basic) solution

The body's goal: maintaining a stable body fluid pH

Just as the body must constantly control its levels of blood sugar, sodium, potassium, calcium, and magnesium, it must also maintain its H+ ion concentration within a very narrow range. As is the case with sodium and potassium (see XXL Syndrome, published by the same edition), a correct concentration of H+ ions is essential for the cells' normal functioning, as the majority of enzymes, the catalysts for all biological reactions, are very sensitive to it.

Two types of acids, two ways of controlling pH

The main acids generated by our bodies are of two types: carbonic acid (H_2CO_3) and non-carbonic acid.

Every day, the digestion of sugars and fats generates carbonic gas (CO_2). Although CO_2 is not an acid, it combines with water to form carbonic acid (H_2CO_3). As a result, if CO_2 were not eliminated by the lungs through respiration, there would be an accumulation of acids in the blood. Therefore, respiration is one of the main ways the body regulates its acid-base balance.

Non-carbonic acids are mainly derived from protein metabolism. Proteins are made of sulfur amino acids such as methionine and cysteine, which form sulfuric acid (H_2SO_4) when oxidized. These H+ ions are eliminated by the kidneys in the urine. Proteins also provide phosphorus, which is a potential source of phosphoric acid.

pH in action

Blood can only tolerate tiny fluctuations in its acidity, whereas tissue and urine pH may reveal larger fluctuations.
Ideal pH values for the human body are:

• 7.3 to 7.4 for extracellular fluid, particularly in lymph, spinal and brain fluid, synovial fluid in the joints, and aqueous humor;

• 7.36 to 7.42 in arterial blood;

• 7.2 to 7.3 for intracellular fluid, particularly in blood and tissue cells;

• 1.2 to 3 in the stomach;

• 7.8 to 8 in the pancreatic juice;

• 6.5 to 7.4 in the saliva;

• 6.5 to 7.5 in the urine.

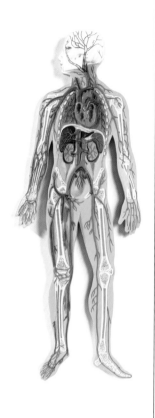

The acid-base balance in our blood

The optimal blood pH value is 7.4, which means that blood is slightly alkaline.

The pH of arterial blood is normally 7.4, while that of venous blood and interstitial fluid is 7.36.
Despite a significant acid burden produced by the food we ingest, the pH of our blood remains remarkably stable, with only tiny variations: the normal range varies only from 7.37 to 7.43. When the blood pH is below 7.37, this is referred to as acidosis, and when the pH is above 7.43, this is referred to as alkalosis. When the blood pH falls outside of this normal range, the patient's health is in serious danger (see inset).

Fortunately, these significant dysfunctions are very rare, because there are several physiological safety nets that constantly maintain blood pH within a normal range. We have already discussed the role of the lungs and kidneys in this area, and the blood buffer system is another control system.

A pH that is too high or too low is a real danger

- If the pH is equal or less than 6.95 (acidosis), there is a risk of coma with cardiac arrest and possibly death;
- If the pH reaches or is greater than 7.7 (alkalosis), there is a risk of tetanic seizures and convulsions which may lead to death.

What does this mean?

A "buffer" solution is a solution made up of two elements, which is able to prevent extreme fluctuations in the pH. A buffer acts by binding to H+ ions when the pH decreases, and releasing H+ ions when the pH increases.

Thus, adding acidic substances to a buffer solution has almost no impact on its pH. Our body has several buffers. The first is the carbonic acid/sodium bicarbonate buffer system. However, there are many others (see inset). Together, these buffer systems aid the body in maintaining a stable pH in its body fluids.

When the balance is disturbed

If one of the regulation systems becomes deficient or, more commonly, if our diet is regularly imbalanced (too many acidifying foods, not enough alkalizing foods), tiny pH variations occur, which will disturb the metabolism, causing waste to accumulate in the body.

First of all, some information on blood pH

Our cells' functioning probably depends more on intracellular fluid pH than on that of extracellular fluid. Yet, the pH of extracellular fluid (blood and lymph) has an impact on intracellular pH, even if the two types of fluid are often very different. Consequently, it is generally assumed that any acid-base imbalance results from an acid-base imbalance in the extracellular fluid.

Any disturbance in the acid-base balance, no matter how slight, will lead to symptoms, such as fatigue, muscle or joint pain, fragile bones, kidney stones, hypertension, diabetes, weight gain… this is not a complete list, and we will see that a number of changes will occur at the cellular level, which will provoke or worsen these problems.

When acidosis becomes chronic

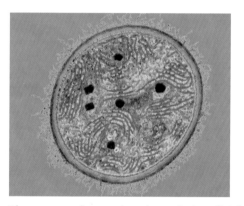

Although significant fluctuations in the acid-base balance are rare, chronic acidosis is much more common. This is a direct consequence of changes in our dietary habits, and the latent acidification of our body is a consequence of our modern lifestyle.

As we have seen, in order for all of our cells to function optimally, it is imperative that the pH of our biological fluids remains within a certain range. The enzymes that catalyze the majority of biological reactions depend on this stability in order to perform. To compensate for any excessive acidity, the body has several different systems to control and regulate the pH: the lungs, kidneys, blood buffer system, etc.

Constipation, a consequence of an acid-base imbalance

If pH conditions are not met in even a tiny section of our digestive tract, digestive juices cannot carry out their function properly: food digestion is incomplete. Thus, when there is too much acidity at the beginning of the small intestine, especially around the duodenum, the proteins and lipids are not digested completely. As a result, these materials are broken down too late, particularly in the colon. This disturbs the fermentation processes which generally take place in this part of the digestive tract, and leads to a putrefaction process, resulting in constipation and bloating, as well as the production of very strong-smelling stools.

The problem is that these systems are not always enough. For example, the kidneys' ability to eliminate H+ ions is limited, and decreases with age. On the other hand, if our diet tends to be very acidifying (too many acidifying foods and not enough alkalizing foods), and the acids generated by our food intake exceed our body's neutralizing capacities, this results in a latent and chronic acidification of our tissues. This chronic acidification is damaging as it hampers vital processes in the heart and in each of our individual cells.

ATPases

Membranous ATPases are a class of enzymes which play a role in cells' energy metabolism. These enzymes "generate" energy flow within the cells. One of these, called ATP synthase, is capable of producing more than 100kg of ATP per day (ATP is the energy reserve molecule in our cells). To this end, it requires optimal pH conditions inside as well as outside the cells. If these conditions are not respected, ATP synthesis cannot occur properly. A latent acidosis thus leads to an energy deficiency within the cells. Several studies have revealed that acidosis leads to a decrease in cellular energy expenditure, while alkalosis stimulates this expenditure. These effects on energy metabolism have been observed in humans.

A slight acid-base imbalance may lead to a vicious cycle, which causes an energy deficiency in our cells. It leads to a slowing down of the cells, and a metabolic block.

pH has an impact on...

• **Immunity**, as antibodies need optimal pH conditions in order to develop and efficiently neutralize antigens;

• **Tissue oxygenation**, as red blood cells need to develop in optimal pH conditions in order to carry oxygen and deliver it throughout the body (hemoglobin's affinity for oxygen is optimal).

Our diet is at the center of the acid-base balance

Our body's acid-base balance depends largely on our diet. More specifically, this balance is strongly conditioned by the "acidic" or "alkaline" nature of the minerals found in our diet.

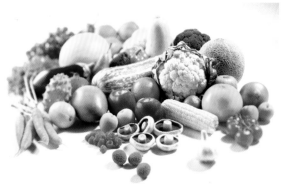

When digestion is completed, nearly all the foods have generated acids and bases in the blood and extracellular fluid.

-Foods that tend to generate more acids than bases are referred to as **acidifying** or "acid-producing" foods. This is particularly the case for foods containing animal proteins (meat, fish, eggs, and shellfish), which generate strong acids, such as hydrochloric acid, sulfuric acid, phosphoric acid, or even uric acid, to name just a few…

Milk and dairy products (yogurt, cheese, etc) contain amino acids which all produce acids to varying degrees. Other notable acid producers include grains, whether or not they are refined.

- Foods that tend to generate more bases than acids are known as **alkalizing** foods. This is particularly the case for fruits and vege-

A good reason to go light on the salt

Chemically speaking, table salt is sodium chloride, and its chemical formula is NaCl. It contains 60% chlorine (Cl) and 40% sodium (Na). (The symbol Na comes from the Latin word for "sodium", natrium). Because of the presence of chlorine, table salt is acidifying. This is why I recommend not salting your food, eating less ready-made meals, and consuming less bread.

tables, although there are certain exceptions. Potatoes (preferably organic), broccoli, and chestnuts are among the most alkalizing foods, as are most leafy green vegetables and tubers.

Finally, there are foods that have no influence on the acid-base balance. They do not increase the acid or alkaline burden, and are neutral. These foods include oils (olive, rapeseed, etc), and refined sugar.

Acidifying or alkalizing, what is the difference ?

A food's acidity depends partly on its mineral balance. It can depend on the quality and quantity of the minerals that it contains. Minerals can be classified into two categories, according to their effect on the body's pH:

-"Acidifying" minerals, which represent chlorine (Cl), sulfur (S), and phosphorus (P), and mainly come from animal proteins and grains;

-"Alkalizing" minerals, the most important of which include potassium (K), calcium (Ca), magnesium (Mg), and sodium (Na), which mainly come from vegetable-based foods.

Change course

Anthony Sebastian, a researcher at the University of San Francisco and renowned specialist in this field, believes that "changing the way we eat can restore the basic makeup of our bodies".

The balance slides toward acidity

If we take a look at acid production on one hand, and alkaline production on the other in our Western diet, we can conclude that the balance slides towards acidity. The Western diet generates an excess of hydrogen ions, with an average of 50mmol.

Pral index

Acidic foods do not necessarily taste sour. These are two different concepts, and we shall discover the reasons why.

As the important factor is the degree of acidity obtained at the end of the digestion process, testing the pH of a slice of meat or a section of a clementine that has just been peeled is of little interest. It would be much more insightful to test the pH of urine or stool after the food has been digested. Of course, this is not very practical! Fortunately, we have the clever invention of Dr. Thomas Remer, an expert in the acid-base balance. While working at the Research Institute for Child Nutrition in Dortmund, Germany, he developed a food rating system referred to as the Pral index (an abbreviation for Potential Renal Acid Load).

This index, expressed in milliequivalents (mEq), allows us to estimate the acid burden of food, based on the assessment of acid and alkaline minerals contained in 100g of this food. As all the minerals are not absorbed in a similar manner by our intestines, the Pral food index must take the absorption coefficient of each element into account.

In short, the Pral food index adds acid minerals and subtracts alkaline minerals. If the final result is more than zero, the food is said to be acidifying. Contrarily, if the final figure is negative, the food is said to be alkalizing. If the figure is zero, the food is considered neutral.

Pral indexes of differents kinds of food

Fats	
Butter	0.6
Margarine	-0.5
Olive oil	0.0
Sunflower oil	**- 0.5**

Fish	
Trout	10.8
Cod	7.1
Herring	7.0
Haddock	**6.8**

Grains	
White bread	3.7
Cornflakes	6.0
Egg pasta	6.4
Oats	10.7
Brown rice	12.5
White rice	4.6
White flour	6.9
Whole-wheat flower	8.2
Whole-wheat bread	**1.8**

Meat	
Beef	7.8
Chicken	8.7
Pork	7.9
Salami	11.8
Turkey	9.9
Veal	9.0
Hot dogs	**6.7**

Dairy products	
Camembert	14.6
Cheddar	26.4
Gouda	18.6
Parmesan	34.2
Fruit-flavored yogurt	1.2
Vanilla ice cream	**0.6**

Eggs	
Chicken eggs	8.2

Sweets	
Cake	3.7
Milk chocolate	2.4
Sucre blanc	-0.1
Honey	-0.3
Marmalade	**-1.5**

Drinks	
Lagger beer	0.9
Coca-Cola	0.4
Tea	-0.3
Hot chocolate	-0.4
Grape juice	-1.0
Dry white wine	-1.2
Coffee	-1.4
Apple juice	-2.2
Red wine	-2.4
Lemon juice	-2.5
Tomato juice	-2.8
Orange juice	**-2.9**

Fresh fruits	
Watermelon	-1.9
Apple	-2.2
Strawberry	-2.2
Peach	-2.4
Pineapple	-2.7
Orange	-2.7
Pear	-2.9
Cherry	-3.6
Kiwi	-4.1
Apricot	-4.8
Banana	-5.5
Blackcurrant	-6.5
Grapes	**-21.0**

Dry fruits	
Nut	6.8
Hazelnuts	**-2.8**

Legumes	
Lentis	3.5
Peas	1.2
Green beans	**-3.1**

Vegetables	
Asparagus	-0.4
Cucumber	-0.8
Broccoli	-1.2
Mushrooms	-1.4
Onions	-1.5
Leek	-1.8
Lettuce	-2.5
Tomato	-3.1
Eggplant	-3.4
Radish	-3.7
Cauliflower	-4.0
Potatoe	-4.0
Zucchini	-4.6
Carrot	-4.9
Celery	-5.2
Spinach	**-14.0**

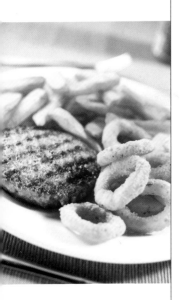

Our modern diet is highly acidifying

Because of our modern lifestyle, we consume foods that generate acids in our bodies. This can lead to chronic acidosis which is damaging for our health. Today, we are well aware of what foods are acidifying.

What are the drawbacks of modern life?

Today, people in industrialized countries tend to eat tremendous quantities of refined grains and animal proteins. They consume large amounts of salty or sweet products, ready-made dishes, and snack constantly. The majority of these foods are highly acidifying. The situation is worsened by the fact that the consumption of fruit and vegetables, which are alkalizing, has plateaued or even dropped off, with the exception of potatoes. The imbalance is striking. The acid burden that our bodies must cope with has progressively increased. It is not neutralized by alkalizing foods, and is directly responsible for numerous health problems, resulting in excessive human and financial costs.

An obvious but worrying situation

To summarize our current situation, we consume:

• Too much salt, which generates acids in our body;

• Too many grains, particularly refined grains, i.e. "empty" grains which contain very few micronutrients and without exception generate acids. Grains alone account for approximately 40% of the daily acid burden produced by our modern Western diet. Grains are found

Man was not made for acidosis

For millions of years, humans genetically evolved to thrive in a very basic environment. Our organs and complex machinery react negatively to certain modern foods, as is proven by the diabetes, osteoporosis and obesity epidemics all around us.

everywhere, throughout the day: from breakfast cereals to white bread, from pasta to the unavoidable pizzas and pies, we want to have our industrially-produced cake and eat it too…

• Too much meat, too many cold cuts, and ready-made meals containing meat products. Our (bad) habit of choosing meat should not make us forget that meat produces strong acids which can overwork our kidneys when they try to eliminate them. On a side note, meat also contains high levels of saturated fat, which is harmful to our arteries;

• Too much milk and too many dairy products: milk is moderately acidifying, while cheese and yogurt are highly acidifying.

The following substances and conditions increase the risk of acidosis :

- Table salt, because chlorine produces hydrochloric acid;
- Animal proteins and grains, because their sulfur-based amino acids generate sulfuric acid;
- Methanol, the type of alcohol found in bourbon, whisky, and cognac;
- Aspirin;
- Diabetes, kidney disease, and age, as the kidneys gradually lose the ability to eliminate acids.

When did the acid-base imbalance begin?

Since the first agricultural evolution, 10,000 years ago, our diets have steadily become acidifying. This trend has worsened over the past century, as we consume the same amount of grains but more meat, dairy products, and salt.

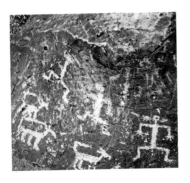

Today, our diet is far more acidifying than that of our grandparents, who themselves could have taken some lessons about nutrition from their ancestors. No one can deny that our dietary habits have undergone a real revolution during the past 30 years, but lifestyles and diets were already being shaken up at the start of the Industrial Age during the 19th century. The true dietary revolution, however, dates back to the Neolithic Age, about 10,000 years ago!

The Neolithic Revolution

Before the Neolithic Age, humans were nomads who gathered fruit, vegetables, roots, and mushrooms; hunted, fished, and scavenged. Their diet was therefore mainly plant-based and rich in vitamins and minerals. The meat that they consumed also contained more muscle and was leaner than what we eat today! Moreover, as all mammals were undomesticated, humans obviously did not consume the milk of other species. As humans gradually became more sedentary and living conditions more secure, birth rates increased, as did the need for readily available food.

The first traces of this shift, which dates back approximately 10,000 years, can be found in an area on the map known as the Fertile Crescent, modern-day Israel, Jordan, and Lebanon. Here, humans found large amounts of wild grains and legumes, which were easy to cultivate, thanks to the region's mild climate. Some 1,500 years later, humans began farming animals which were easy to capture, such as sheep, goats, pigs, and cows. Agriculture and animal husbandry continued to evolve, and eventually exploded with the food industry of the 20th century.

In short, one can say that less than 10,000 years ago (or 5,000 years before the construction of the Great Pyramid of Giza), the following occurred:

• Grains, which were previously almost unheard of, began to constitute a major source of sulfur and, consequently, acidity;

• More meat was available for consumption, as animals were farmed;

• Milking other mammals became easier, thus humans began to consume this milk;

• As a result of animal husbandry and agriculture becoming a full-time occupation, less gathering foods such as fruit, berries, legumes, nuts, roots, mushrooms, etc., which are rich in alkalizing compounds, were consumed.

The prehistoric diet

American researchers estimated that by reverting back to the prehistoric diet of our ancestors, which was rich in plant-based products and non-grain foods, we could reestablish our body's fundamental basic character. Contemporary hunter-gatherers have maintained a lifestyle which protects them from excess acidity. During the 1960's, the urine of a tribe from New Guinea was measured and the results showed a urine pH between 7.5 and 9, thanks to a diet rich in potassium bicarbonate. What an example to our modern society!

The negative effects of modern foods

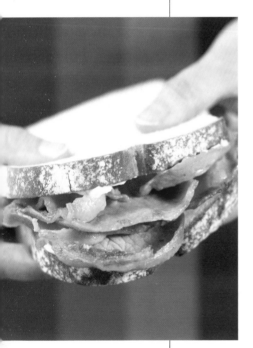

Acidifying foods, typical of our modern era, are directly responsible for the acidification of our body, which has numerous harmful effects, and puts the body at risk for other problems. Some of these risks are well-known, others less so... Here is an overview.

- The high content of saturated fat in meat-based foods and dairy products expose the consumer to a greater risk of developing cardiovascular disease. To this, we can add the traces of antibiotics and chemical substances administered to livestock, as well as the intense stress that modern farming and slaughtering conditions exert on the animals... We should also not forget about the current wastefulness of intensive farming, which applies to the foods or farmland used for feeding livestock.

- Due to the growing suspicions regarding the so-called benefits of milk and dairy products, we should take care to consume them in moderation. Due to its content in hormones (estrogens; progesterone), growth factors, proteins and allergenic lactose, an excessive consumption of dairy (four to five servings per day, which is quite common today), will likely increase one's risk of developing chronic diseases.

- Our modern diet, compared to that of our Paleolithic ancestors, is clearly lacking potassium. For the vast majority of human history, we consumed only small amounts of salt (2g of sodium per day) and large amounts of potassium, approximately 12g per day. With the discovery of the usefulness of salt in preserving foods, came the discovery of its taste-enhancing property. Since then, the dietary sodium/potassium ratio has gradually become inversed. Today, modern humans consume 10g of salt per day and only 2g of potassium daily: two to four times more sodium than potassium.

- The omega-6/omega-3 ratio has also evolved in the wrong direction, essentially due to the fact that sunflower oil (rich in omega-6) has become widely used in cooking during the last few decades.

- Last on the list of culprits is sugar. Those individuals who do not have a sweet tooth are few and far between. Sugar is found everywhere and we consume astronomical amounts of it. Though food labels on ready-made products do mention sugar content, many people also have a habit of adding sugar to coffee, yogurt or grapefruit. Sugar makes us vulnerable to dental cavities, excess weight, diabetes, and other hazards of our modern times.

Salt + sugar + fat : an explosive cocktail

According to the New York Times, Americans consume on average 31% more packaged food than fresh food. Examples of this include frozen pizza, microwave dinners, and sweet or salty snacks. According to Dr. James A. Howenstine, Americans are world leaders when it comes to soda consumption, drinking 3 quarts per week per capita. According to the United States Department of Agriculture, between 1909 and 2001, American cheese consumption per capita increased by 800%. Today, over half of the cheese consumed in the United States is found in commercially manufactured and prepared foods. The overabundance of highly processed, salty, sweet, fatty, and **highly acidifying** foods supports the progression of diseases such as cardiovascular disease, osteoporosis, diabetes, cancer, and obesity, the latter affecting more than 30% of all Americans, according to the United States Center for Disease Control.

Reestablish your acid-base balance for better health

Our diet, which should be composed of 80% of alkalizing foods and 20% of acidifying foods, as it was before the Neolithic Revolution, has been completely turned upside down. Acidifying foods, such as meat and grains, have become the front-runners in our diets.

How can you get back to this balance?

It is almost impossible to revert back to our ancestors' diet, but it is possible to get closer to it. Generally speaking, you should compensate the consumption of **one portion of an acidifying food with at least two portions of alkalizing foods.**

It is almost impossible to revert back to our ancestors' diet, but it is possible to get closer to it. Generally speaking, you should compensate the consumption of one portion of an acidifying food with at least two portions of alkalizing foods. Acidifying foods are usually:

- Dairy products, especially cheese, the record being held by parmesan, which has a Pral index of 34;

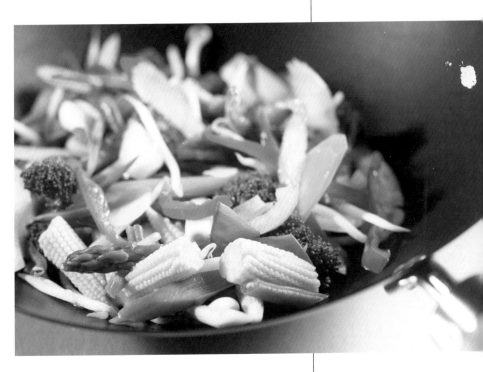

- Meat and cold cuts, with a record Pral index for rabbit and high indexes for poultry;

- Fish, shellfish, and seafood, mussels and crayfish having the highest indexes;

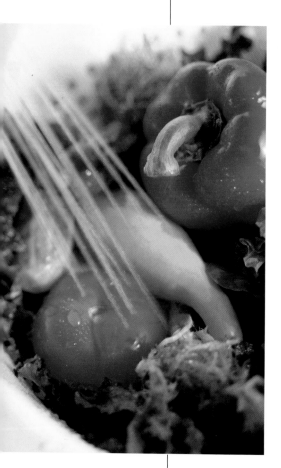

- Grains, with a record index for whole-wheat rice, followed by oats.

On the other end of the spectrum are alkalizing foods, including fruit and vegetables, tea, herbal teas, and even wine. The most alkalizing vegetables, which are those that counteract chronic acidosis most effectively, are spinach, parsley, and celery. The most alkalizing fruits are dried fruits: figs, raisins, etc.

Therefore, for each portion of cheese, meat, or grains, eat two servings of vegetables, legumes, or fruit.

Water to the rescue!

Mineral water can also fight against the body's acidification if it is rich in bicarbonates. This is generally true for sparkling water. This type of water is usually rich in sodium, and more importantly, the sodium is bound to bicarbonates and not chloride ions. In this form, sodium does not cause hypertension, contrary to what many doctors believe. Some reports have warned against mineral water with a high sodium content, such as Vichy Springs, Lithia Springs, and Montclair, as they are not recommended for patients suffering from high blood pressure, or heart and kidney insufficiency. However, these reports do not take into account that in mineral waters, sodium is generally bound to bicarbonate. In this case, sodium has no harmful effects on the heart, lungs or blood pressure. In fact, several studies have revealed rather beneficial effects.

One can also easily replace classic sodium- and chloride-based table salt with a sodium- and potassium-based table salt. These types of salt can be found in pharmacies and health stores.

« Genetically speaking, our bodies are identical to those of the late Paleolithic Age, approximately 20,000 years ago. The introduction of agriculture and animal husbandry, some 10,000 years ago, and the Industrial Revolution, approximately 200 years ago, introduced new dietary pressure to which it was impossible to adapt in such a short space of time. There is, therefore, an obvious discrepancy between our diet and the diet for which our genes are adapted». N.J. Mann, Australian nutritionist, 2004.

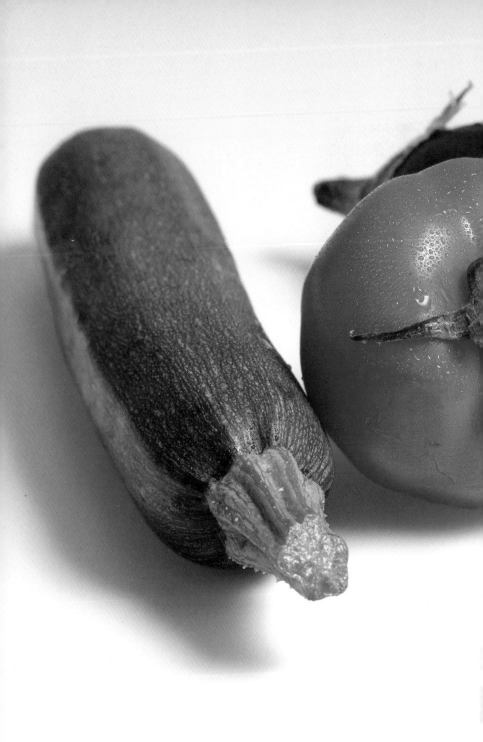

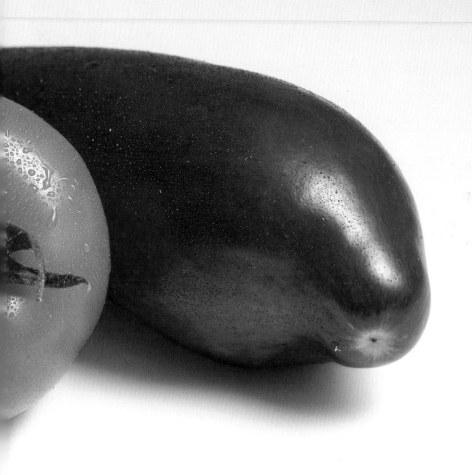

THE CONSEQUENCES
OF AN ACID-BASE
IMBALANCE

Osteoporosis, a misdiagnosed and poorly treated epidemic

Osteoporosis affects eight million women and two million men in the United States. There have been many attempts to prevent this frequently misdiagnosed epidemic with inappropriate and ineffective recommendations.

The osteoporosis epidemic

Osteoporosis is a disease that affects the bones, and particularly occurs in postmenopausal women. It is characterized by a loss in bone mass and a deterioration of the bones' microarchitecture. The occurrence of osteoporosis increases with age: 10% in women under the age of 60, 20% in women under the age of 65, and 40% in women over 75 years of age have osteoporosis. In the United States, eight million women are thought to be affected by this generalized skeletal demineralization which increases the risk of fractures, especially femoral head fractures, which occur in approximately 297,000 people every year. Wrist fractures – a warning sign of osteoporosis from the age of 55– concern 397,000 people. Lastly, 547,000 new spine fractures (or spinal com-

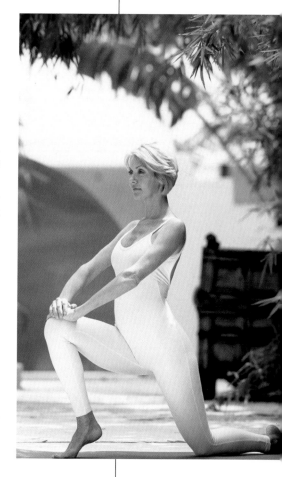

pression fractures) are diagnosed in the United States every year, while the actual number of these fractures, which often go unnoticed, is estimated to be much higher. One out of five patients who were able to walk prior to their hip fracture will require long-term care. Both hip and spine fractures are associated with a risk of death.

More dairy products are not the solution

As a solution for osteoporosis, health authorities in all developed countries, which are also the countries with the highest rates of osteoporosis, encourage the population to increase their consumption of calcium, usually from animal products, such as milk and dairy. The

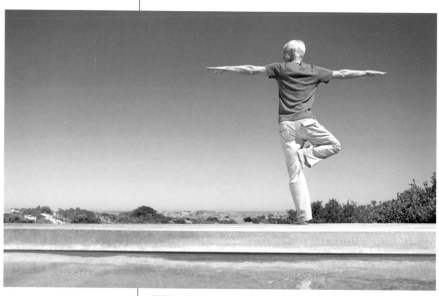

USDA recommends consuming two to three servings of dairy products per day. In reality, this strategy is not providing any results. The World Health Organization (WHO) has come to the conclusion that the countries which consume the largest amount of dairy products and dietary calcium are actually the most affected by the femoral head fracture epidemic. On the other hand, countries with little or no dairy calcium consumption encounter the smallest amount of femoral head fractures. In order to qualify the situation, WHO coined the term the "calcium paradox". Moreover, epidemiological and clinical studies conducted on a homogenous population group have not yet shown any results suggesting that children, adolescents, and adults who consume more dairy products suffer fewer fractures than others.

The most likely reason for the fact that dairy products do not prevent osteoporosis is that bone health depends more on your acid-base balance than on the quantity of calcium you consume.

A very costly epidemic

The number of femoral head fractures linked to the population's aging may nearly quadruple world-wide between now and 2050. According to the medical journal The Lancet, which published this prediction in June 2006, this would mean that the number of these fractures would increase from 1.7 million in 1990 to 6.3 million. The study's authors were concerned about the health costs that this epidemic will lead to. The majority of people ignore this danger, which could be avoided by a sufficient dietary intake of calcium, regular physical activity, and in some cases, specific drugs. In the United States, fractures related to osteoporosis were responsible for approximately $19 billion in costs. By the year 2025, it is estimated that this figure will be $25.3 billion.

Osteoporosis, an acid-base imbalance disease

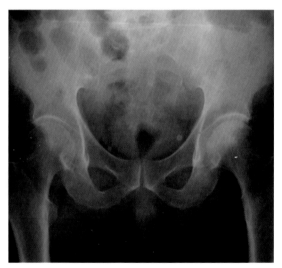

The prevention of osteoporosis entails, first of all, an alkalizing diet which protects bone calcium.

Acidosis and decalcification

Osteoporosis, which is known as the "brittle bone disease", is also a typical disease in developed countries. This condition can be partly accounted for by the consequences of an acid-base imbalance. 10,000 years ago, when humans became sedentary and began consuming tremendous amounts of grains, animal products, and salt as nutrition, our diets became acidifying. This trend has worsened over the course of the last century.

Our diet has plunged our bodies into a chronic state of acidosis, causing our bones to suffer. There is a simple explanation for this: in order to neutralize excess acid, the body takes citrate and bicarbonate from the bones. As these compounds are bound to calcium, calcium is excreted in the urine and is subsequently missing in the bones.

This mechanism has been misunderstood for a very long time already, even longer than suspected, as the first mention of it dates back to 1880. In 1920, Henry Clapp Sherman from Columbia University established that excess amounts of animal proteins increase the excretion of bone calcium, a fact that has been proven repeatedly. For example, if the consumption of animal proteins is doubled (from 35 to 78g per day), the amount of calcium excreted in the urine increases by 50%.

A solution: an alkalizing diet

The most effective way of preventing osteoporosis pro-bably consists of inducing a light state of alkalosis in your body by adjusting your dietary habits: consuming less salt, animal proteins, and grains – all of which have an acidifying effect –, and eating more fruit and vege-tables, which provide alkalizing elements, such as potas-sium salts. Several studies have also shown an improvement in bone density in women who consume more fruit and vegetables, or who take potassium bicar-bonate. When the average daily potassium consumption of a group of menopausal women was increased from 2.3 to 5.4g, the level of calcium in the urine decreased by 64mg. This corresponds to theoretical "savings" on calcium requirements of approximately 300mg per day. With this type of diet, it is unnecessary to gorge oneself on calcium.

How much calcium?

As Western diets are high in salt and animal proteins which eliminate calcium, we need 800 to 1 000mg of calcium per day. We calculated that if you consume less than 5g of salt and less than 20g of animal proteins per day – the equivalent of a 100g steak –, you will only need 400mg of calcium in order to keep your bones in good health. Similar figures can be obtained by eating fruit and vegetables, or slightly less grains.

Other prevention factors

In addition to an alkalizing diet, you must make sure to:

- Engage in regular physi-cal activity;
- Consume sufficient amounts of omega-3 contained in nuts, rape-seed oil, oily fish, or fish oil capsules;
- Get enough vitamin D by taking supplements which provide at least 1,000 IU per day, between October and April in the Northern hemisphere;
- Consume enough vita-min K (leafy vegetables, spinach, or supplements).

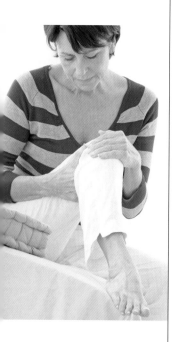

When joints become painful

Gout and arthrosis are two rheumatoid diseases that chronic acidosis makes us vulnerable to.

In some people, excess acidity caused by their diet can lead to what is commonly known as gout. Acute bouts of gout are particularly painful, but keeping to an alkalizing diet can put an end to them quickly.

Uric acid is to blame...

Carnivorous animals produce an enzyme called uricase, which eliminates uric acid generated by the breaking down of purines– the components in meat. Sometimes, humans also consume large amounts of meat, however, they do not produce uricase. Therefore, we are at risk of overproducing uric acid. When we have a high-protein diet, which is highly acidifying, uric acid levels increase. Beyond a specific pH threshold, uric acid begins to crystallize (the solubility of uric acid decreases with the pH level). These crystals are deposited in our joints, tissues, and also in the kidneys, which leads to the formation of kidney stones– a risk not to be taken lightly, as one in ten people will develop kidney stones at least once in his or her lifetime.

Gout: an age-old problem

Gout has been recognized since ancient times, where it was known as "the kings' disease", as it predominantly affected people who ate and drank "well". Gout is indeed linked to diet, particularly to some foods with high

Gout affects more men than women

Gout occurs more frequently in men than in women, which suggests that apart from our diet's acid burden, hormonal factors also play a role. Gout becomes more frequent with age.

levels of purines, which produce uric acid. Gout occurs either when the body generates too much uric acid (due to an excessively acidifying diet), or when uric acid is not completely excreted in the urine (the kidneys are not fulfilling their function as acid-base balance regulators). Gout frequently occurs in the big toes, but also in the ankles, knees, wrists, and fingers. While it may remain latent for a long time, gout may also affect relatively young people around the age of 30 to 40 years.

Purine-rich foods

Purine content (mg)

Cow's liver (100g)	360
Sardines (100g)	345
Calf's liver (100g)	260
Chicken liver (100g)	243
Trout (100g)	200
Boletus mushrooms (100g)	184
Chicken breast, with skin (100g)	175
Salmon (100g)	170
Cooked ham (100g)	130
Roast beef (100g)	110

Putting yourself at risk for rheumatism!

Acid crystals which have accumulated in the body act like grains of sand and lead to the deterioration of joints. Joints become less supple and are riddled with painful inflammations.

The first line of treatment for gout entails adopting an alkalizing diet rich in plant products. You must reduce your consumption of animal proteins and alcohol considerably. On the other hand, it is essential that you drink plenty of water (more than two liters of water per day).

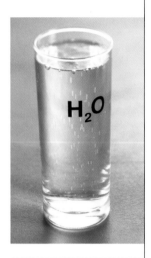

H_2O

"Stones" in the kidneys

Renal calculus (kidney stones) stems from the Latin calculus, which means "stone", and is caused by the crystallization of chemical substances found in the urine. By adhering to each other, crystals form a stone (or calculus) which may be the size of a grain of sand or... a golf ball! Most of these stones are formed in the kidneys.

The plan of action for preventing kidney stones

Whatever the type of stone, these six rules should be followed:
- Drink at least a half a gallon of water per day;
- Avoid strict vegetarian diets;
- Avoid diets rich in animal proteins;
- Limit your salt intake;
- Eat sufficient amounts of vegetables and legumes;
- Avoid exposure to toxins (pesticides, solvents, and excessive amounts of painkillers like tylenol).

As we have already mentioned, kidney stones may result from the crystallization of uric acid, which comes from our diet, or the purines that our body's cells reject when the urine's pH is too acidic. However, in other cases, kidney stones consist of calcium oxalate, a combination of oxalic acid and calcium. Once again, diet, plays a role, as large amounts of calcium are found in the urine when the body is acidified (see page 32 on osteoporosis). This calcium can then be captured by oxalic acid from foods, such as sorrel (with the highest content), rhubarb, spinach, chocolate, as well as tea. The latter also contains purines...

The solution: alkalize urine

In order to prevent the formation of uric acid stones, drinking enough liquids so as to produce at least a half a gallon of urine per day is recommended. You should change your diet so that your urine's pH level is always between 6.2 and 6.5.

Chronically tired

While there are clear symptoms of metabolic acidosis (a severe disorder), chronic acidosis does not manifest itself in any spectacular way. Most of the time, this latent imbalance goes completely unnoticed. It is exhaustion and persistent fatigue which provide us with the necessary clues.

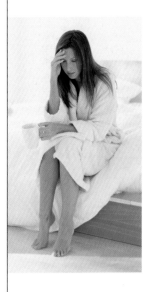

Chronic acidosis in the tissues and body fluids propels the body into a vicious cycle, leading to a state of energy failure in the cells, and consequently, slowed cellular activity and metabolic block. When each cell's metabolism slows down, the entire body struggles to find the necessary energy to move and think. Muscle cells do not contract properly anymore, nerve cells are run down, you feel tired, have a slower reaction speed, are sluggish, and irritable: extreme lethargy takes over.

Athletic people should pay attention to their acid-base balance!

Everyone has suffered from aches and pains after intense physical exercise at least once in their life. These are signs of the accumulation of lactic acid in your muscles. Lactic acid is produced when you work your muscles, and is usually gradually eliminated as it is being produced. Unfortunately, it cannot be eliminated fast enough when you suffer from chronic acidosis (cells are in a state of energy failure, tissues are not supplied with sufficient oxygen), which frequently results in aches and pains.

On a side note, the main alkalizing minerals, such as calcium and potassium, are crucial for sports performance, recovery, and muscle development. They play a fundamental role in the contractility and excitability of muscles. Another reason to maintain a good acid-base balance.

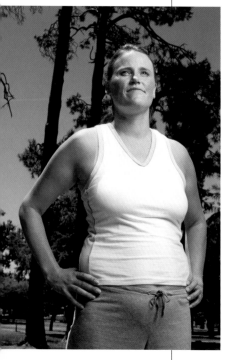

From insulin resistance to being overweight

Although being overweight is not a recent problem, it is nonetheless a public health concern. Too many calories, not enough exercise, defective genes... there is no doubt that the excess weight "epidemic", that is currently taking over the world, can be ascribed to a combination of several factors. Chronic acidosis is one of the culprits.

Weight is a matter of balance. In order to keep your weight constant and reasonable, you have to maintain a balance between your energy input (food consumption) on one hand, and energy expenditure [energy required by the body in order to function (approximately 70%) + energy spent on physical activity (approximately 30%)] on the other.

If you consume more calories than you use, your body must deal with the excess calories by storing them as fat. If your diet is highly acidifying, this is even more likely to happen.

Acidosis disrupts hormone levels

Recent research has shown that chronic acidosis brought about by a diet rich in protein and low in potassium

The risks of obesity

- Obesity increases the risk of stroke.
- The risk of heart attack is 150% higher in overweight individuals, and twice as high in obese individuals.

salts leads to increased levels of the stress hormone cortisol. This hormone is likely to cause an increase in abdominal fat, which in turn can lead to insulin resistance. This downward spiral can be disastrous, as insulin resistance carries considerable consequences for the body. Over the long term, it leads to a chronically increased insulin level and a host of disturbances which have been named "XXL syndrome", and include obesity, diabetes or prediabetes, heart problems, hypertension, insufficient levels of "good" cholesterol (HDL), increased triglyceride levels, etc.

Heavy figures

A total of 63% of all Americans are overweight or obese. Among youth, this figure is 13%.

Insulin resistance and XXL syndrome*

The history of insulin resistance and XXL syndrome dates back more than 60 years, when researchers began suspecting that insulin plays a key role in certain chronic diseases. Insulin is a hormone which is secreted by the pancreas and released into the blood when we consume carbohydrates (sugars, grains, potatoes, etc.) and, to a lesser degree, when we eat proteins and fats. The carbohydrates we consume are transformed into glucose. The role of insulin is to enable our cells to access blood glucose in order to fulfill the body's needs. This allows our blood glucose level, known as "blood sugar", to remain relatively stable.

When muscle cells (but also liver, body fat, and vascular wall cells) no longer respond to insulin's commands, this is known as insulin resistance. As a result, blood sugar tends to remain high, and the pancreas frantically produces more and more insulin in order to remedy the situation.

* *The XXL Syndrome, Dr Max Rombi, Alpen Editions*

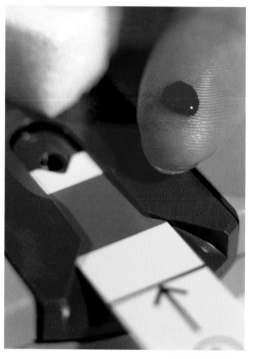

Alkalizing diets and diabetes

Today, diabetes patients benefit from a large number of dietary recommendations, but only few doctors are familiar with the true positive effects that a slightly alkalizing diet has on the disease itself and its complications.

Our Paleolithic ancestors had an alkalizing diet, as they consumed mostly plant products: fruit, vegetables, leaves, roots, tubers, and nuts. This high-potassium diet disappeared 10,000 years ago when humans adopted a sedentary lifestyle. Today, our diet clearly carries an acid burden, as we consume large quantities of grains (acidifying), meat, cold cuts, dairy products, salt, but only small amounts of potassium – four times less than 15,000 to 20,000 years ago.

Our modern diet has obvious effects on interstitial pH, which it decreases, as well as on insulin levels, which results in an increased risk of kidney disease and vascular complications for the more fragile among us: diabetes patients and insulin-resistant individuals, who can be qualified as prediabetics.

In September 2007, a Swedish research team had the idea to compare the effect of two types of diets in insulin-resistant, glucose-intolerant, or diabetic patients: a Mediterranean-like diet and a Paleolithic diet.

Nutritionists often consider the Mediterranean diet to be "ideal", but with its grains and dairy products, it is still acidifying. The Paleolithic diet, on the other hand, is alkalizing: in this study, it consisted of fruit, vegetables, tubers, nuts, eggs, meat, and fish. Results showed that after 12 weeks, blood glucose levels decreased by 7% in the "Mediterranean" group -a respectable result-, but dropped by 26% in the "Paleolithic" group – a spectacular result! Insulin levels also decreased. This study suggests that an alkalizing diet can improve diabetics' and prediabetics' conditions more than a Mediterranean-like diet can. As glucose intolerance increases the risk of peripheral neuropathy in diabetics, a Paleolithic diet may reduce complications.

Chemical sugar damage

The most serious complication of diabetes stems from hemoglobin glycation. Excess glucose in the blood is likely to lead to a certain chemical reaction: the bonding of glucose to hemoglobin in red blood cells. This reaction is called glycation. As a result, red blood cells become less supple, which results in microcirculation problems in the capillaries, notably in the retina, kidneys, and extremities. Glycogen may also bond to insulin, which then becomes inactive. This partially accounts for insulin resistance.

Asthma: an acid-base balance matter

Asthma is accompanied by metabolic acidosis, which can endanger the patient's life. For this reason, acidity regulators are given during severe asthma attacks. However, the prevention of asthma and its complications firstly entail adjusting one's diet.

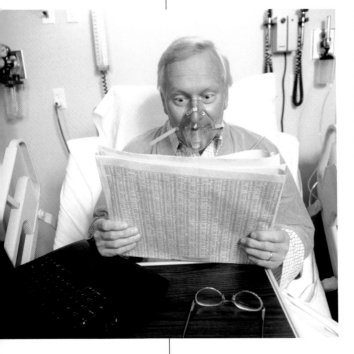

Asthma attacks may turn dramatic and endanger the patient's life and can be a result of metabolic acidosis. Respiratory muscles have to work intensively, and under this strain, they produce excess lactic acid. Moreover, as tissues are lacking oxygen and the volume of blood expelled by the heart is reduced, acidosis is even more severe. It is therefore very important to treat acidosis in these patients. To this effect, potassium bicarbonate is usually administered intravenously in order to reduce bronchial spasms and restore the response of bronchodilators.

Outside of these severe attacks, potassium bicarbonate and magnesium supplements, two factors which treat chronic acidosis, may be administered to asthma patients in combination with an alkalizing diet. Several studies have revealed that asthmatics actually lack potassium, particularly during acute attacks. Researchers therefore recommend administering potassium supplements.

Potassium's enemies

Theophylline is an asthma drug which may deplete potassium in the body. The same can be said for the excessive consumption of caffeine (coffee, tea, and sodas) and salt.

Potassium deficiencies increase the risk of asthma

Studies show that overall, people who only take in small amounts of potassium and magnesium breathe less efficiently than those with the highest intake. Potassium- and magnesium-deficient individuals are also at higher risk of developing asthma. Therefore, if you suffer from respiratory problems, it is very important to consume sufficient amounts of potassium-rich foods, such as fruit, vegetables, and fish. Moreover, magnesium is also useful for maintaining good potassium levels.

Muscle melt-down

With age, the overall muscle mass in our body decreases. While the muscles represent 45% of our body weight at age 30, this number melts down to 27% at age 70. This is a normal aging process, which is, however, accelerated and occurs sooner if your diet is highly acidifying.

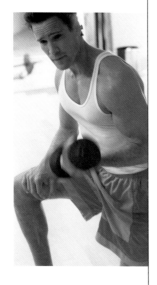

As we explained earlier, one of the major consequences of chronic acidosis is the excessive depletion of calcium in the bones, which is then excreted in the urine, leading to weakened bones. The same process occurs in our muscles. Another way our body neutralizes excess acidity is by binding glutamine (an amino acid) to hydrogen ions $H+$ in order to form ammonium ions $NH4+$, which are then excreted in the urine.

Therefore, in the fight against chronic acidosis, glutamine is used by the body in the same way as calcium. Where in the body is glutamine found? Amino acids are mainly

Our muscles are our best form of health insurance

It cannot be said enough: muscles play a central role in our health. As they are comprised of proteins, our muscle mass is a bulk of proteins which constantly renew themselves by using the amino acids provided by our diet: our body's source of amino acids. This source is **crucial** because it enables us to produce all the proteins that our body needs (hormones, antibodies, etc.). Having healthy muscles is our insurance: it allows us to effectively "repair" ourselves if we suffer injuries, and to defend" ourselves against severe infections. It also allows us to control our blood sugar levels.

found in our muscles (read insert). By encouraging the release of glutamine, chronic acidosis causes the deterioration of muscle proteins. This way, chronic acidosis accelerates the loss in muscle mass.

What happen when we regain our acid-base balance?

Researchers gave potassium bicarbonate, an alkalizing salt, to 14 menopausal women whose diets were acidifying. They noted that this supplement allowed them to effectively treat chronic acidosis, and that the acid production as well as the destruction of muscle proteins decreased. The authors of this study concluded that "by regaining an acid-base balance, the absorption of potassium bicarbonate is high enough to prevent the age-related decrease in muscle mass, and even to repair damage caused by chronic acidosis."

Sufficient muscle mass is important for good health

This means:
- engaging in regular physical activity;
- fighting against chronic acidosis.

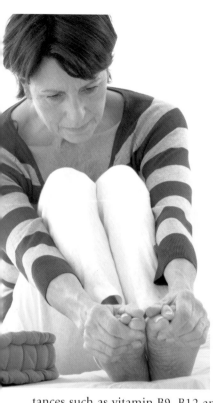

A fungal paradise

The good health of the various bacterial flora in our bodies depends on a good acid-base balance. Too much acidity may cause fungal infections.

We live in symbiosis with a multitude of germs and bacteria. The best example is the bacterial flora inhabiting our intestines. These bacteria are extremely important for our health. Firstly, by acting as a barrier, they prevent most bad bacteria from anchoring themselves in our body. Secondly, they are crucial for our digestion because they ferment certain undigested carbohydrates, thereby producing gas and substances such as vitamin B9, B12 and K, which are beneficial to our health. Lastly, intestinal flora continuously communicate with intestinal cells which control immunity. By communicating with this system, intestinal flora can modify immunity.

The intestines are not the only organ containing bacteria. Each organ has its own bacterial flora. We have oral flora, vaginal flora, pulmonary flora, skin flora, and so on. There is a multitude of germs, of which certain types are dominant in number. These flora are also in harmony with our entire body. However, if the biological equilibrium between the bacteria and their host is disrupted, some of them may become harmful to the body.

When the acid-base balance is disrupted

The biological equilibrium between the bacteria and their host is very fragile. As soon as one of the physiochemical parameters is off-balance, the flora become very sensitive and fragile. As a result, fungi may start developing, become predominant, and cause fungal infections.

- Too much heat and humidity (as when feet are enclosed in shoes) may lead to the growth of fungi of the Candida albicans type between the toes, a condition which is commonly known as athlete's foot.
- An excessively acidic internal body environment may also offset the floral equilibrium. This may cause vaginal yeast infections, thrush (oral candidiasis), certain urinary tract infections, etc.

The solution is to alkalize

By re-establishing an alkaline environment, we can regain the equilibrium between our different flora. By sticking to a diet rich in plant products, which are alkalizing, we can efficiently prevent these problems from recurring.

Down with oral candidiasis!

Oral candidiasis is a condition caused by a fungus (Candida albicans) and affects the digestive tract. In a healthy person, Candida is found in the resident oral flora. The problem is that it is an opportunistic fungus, which means that when the conditions are right, for example, if the host suffers from chronic acidosis, it may become predominant. The result is the appearance of creamy white patches which are more or less spread-out, causing bleeding and burning sensations, and impairing chewing. The solution is washing your mouth out with baking soda. The same applies to the treatment of athlete's foot: powder your feet with baking soda or potassium bicarbonate.

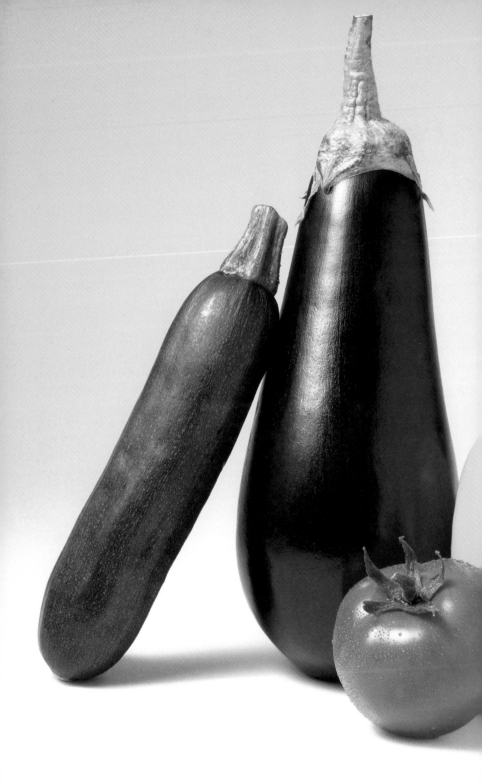

CONTROL
YOUR ACIDITY

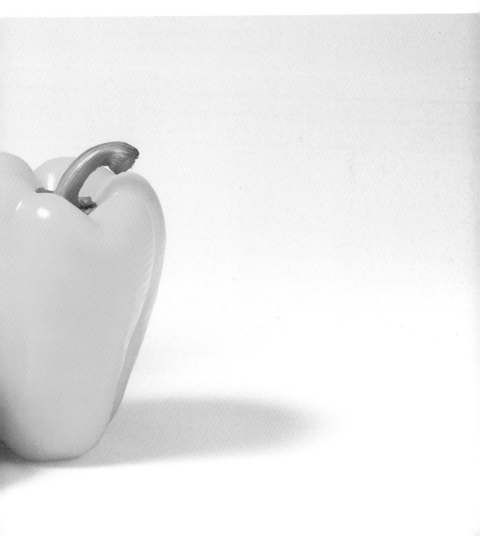

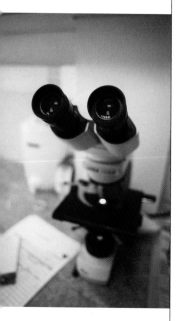

How do I know if I am too acidic?

A simple test can give you information about the acidic or alkaline character of your body, allowing you to take the necessary measures to re-establish a balance.

Blood pH is maintained in a narrow range of 7.35 to 7.45. When your blood pH is low, (a sign of acidosis), the kidneys react by excreting more acid in the urine. Urinary pH decreases until blood pH returns to normal. It may be useful to measure the pH of the urine (or saliva) in order to determine if you need to change your diet. This adjustment may entail taking supplements, such as potassium bicarbonate.

The pH of urine or saliva is measured using strips designed for this purpose. You can find them in pharmacies, health stores, or buy them by mail order. The instructions are simple: dip the strip in a small bottle containing a sample of your urine or saliva.

My pH is too low or too high: should I be worried?

In some cases, an excessively high or low pH may indicate a health problem.

- High pH: may occur if you have a urinary tract infection, emphysema, or impaired kidney function. If your urine is too alkaline, your risk of developing kidney stones made of calcium carbonate, calcium phosphate, or magnesium phosphate, may increase.

- Low pH: may occur if you suffer from emphysema, diabetes, diarrhea, or anorexia. A low pH can increase the risk of kidney stones made of xanthine, cystine, uric acid, or calcium oxalate.

You should test the urine from the second time you urinate during the day, as the urine is often acidic the first time. Test urine from several trips to the bathroom during the course of the day, and calculate the average. Do not wait before dipping the strip into the urine: Bacteria change into urea and ammonia, artificially raising the pH.

In order to analyze your saliva, test several samples during the course of the day, just as it should be done for urine.

How do I interpret the average result?

- pH between 7.0 and 7.5: an optimal result;
- pH <6.0: a sign of acidosis;
- pH >8: a sign alkalosis.

My pH is too low or too high: should I be worried?

In some cases, an excessively high or low pH may indicate a health problem.
- High pH: may occur if you have a urinary tract infection, emphysema, or impaired kidney function. If your urine is too alkaline, your risk of developing kidney stones made of calcium carbonate, calcium phosphate, or magnesium phosphate, may increase.
- Low pH: may occur if you suffer from emphysema, diabetes, diarrhea, or anorexia. A low pH can increase the risk of kidney stones made of xanthine, cystine, uric acid, or calcium oxalate.

The diet that can remedy acidosis

An alkalizing diet is something you can start today. Here are its main principles.

Type of food	Choose	Avoid
Meat	Poultry (chicken, duck, guinea fowl, turkey, goose, etc. skinless), beef, and lamb. Choose lean cuts.	Fatty cuts. Industrially-packaged cold cuts.
Seafood	All fish, especially herring, and salmon; oysters.	Cans of fish in oil. Fish eggs. Deep-fried or stir-fried fish. Smoked fish. Fishsticks.
Eggs	Hard & soft-boiled, sunny-side up, scrambled, in omelets.	Industrially-produced omelets. Eggs in aspic.
Fruit and vegetables	All fresh or frozen vegetables. All fresh fruit. Legumes: peas, butter beans, red kidney beans, broad beans, and soy beans.	Canned vegetables, canned or sachet soup Fruit in syrup. Freeze-dried purée, au gratin style potatoes. Frozen pot pies, French fries. Dried salty and toasted cocktail snacks.
Grains	Almonds and hazelnuts. Multi-grain whole-wheat bread. Whole-wheat rice,	White bread, crustless bread, biscuits. Instant white rice, precooked frozen rice.

Type of food	Choose	Avoid
Grains	wild rice, and basmati rice. Whole-wheat pasta. Sugar-free muesli; oats.	Instant pasta. All sugary and toasted breakfast cereals. Pastries, confectionary and industrially-produced sugary cookies. Crackers. Pizza, quiches, and salty tarts.
Dairy products	Plain yogurt, cheese; cottage cheese.	Industrially-produced cheese. Yogurt and other sweet dairy desserts. Chocolate milk.
Fats, oil-producing plants, seasoning, and condiments	Olive, rapeseed, nut, and soybean oil. Rapeseed margarine. Peanuts, Macadamia nuts, and unsalted pistachios. Garlic, onions, shallots, parsley, basil, tarragon, spring onion, thyme, rosemary, bay leaves, etc.	Lightly salted butter and fresh cream. Solid fat for deep-frying. Bouillon cubes, sauce bases, fish sauce, and industrial soy or teriyaki sauce. Mustard and ketchup. Store-bought salad dressing. Gherkins.
Beverages	Calcium- and magnesium-rich still mineral water. Alkalizing sparkling mineral water. Freshly-squeezed fruit juice or 100% pure fruit juice with no added sugar. Herbal tea. Wine (one to two glasses daily).	Tomato juice. Sodas. **In moderation :** alcohol, coffee, and tea.

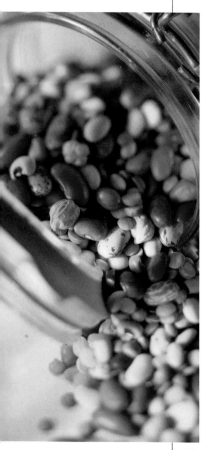

The alkalizing diet in practice

Here is a detailed look at the alkalizing diet recommendations for each food group.

One rule should be kept in mind: for each portion of acidifying foods (offal, meat, dairy products, grains, and some legumes and nuts), you should consume two portions of alkalizing foods (fruit, vegetables, and some types of sparkling mineral water).

Fruit, vegetables, and legumes: at least seven portions daily

Fruit and vegetables should make up the main part of your diet in volume and weight. All fruit and vegetables are beneficial, and you should eat at least seven portions of them daily. Fruit juice can replace a portion, as long as it only replaces one daily portion. One portion of soup counts as one portion of vegetables, providing that it is a home-made soup, and that it is no too strained. Buy seasonal fruit and vegetables.

You can eat at least three portions of legumes weekly. Legumes are moderately acidifying. This is particularly true of tofu (soy), chickpeas, and lentils. However, soy milk, beans, and peas are only slightly acidifying.

Fats and dry oil-producing plants: two to four portions daily

There are no particular remarks to be made about added fats as long as they keep a good balance between fatty acids: rapeseed oil, olive oil, and rapeseed margarine for seasoning; and olive oil, or if necessary, goose fat, for cooking. It is preferable to buy virgin and organic oil. Butter should be used sparingly because it contains saturated fat, and is slightly acidifying.

Oil-producing plants (nuts) are included in this food group. The most acidifying nuts are Brazil nuts, cashew nuts, and Grenoble nuts. The least acidifying are pecans.

Grains: zero to six portions daily

Grains are generally acidifying. This is particularly true for breakfast cereals, pizza, rice cakes, pancakes, croissants, cakes like pound cake, and ladyfingers. Bread is moderately acidifying, as is rice. Only slightly acidifying foods include cookies, fruit tartes, whole-wheat rice, wild rice, gingerbread, and spaghetti.

In order to remedy severe acidosis, you must completely avoid grains for a certain amount of time, or give them up forever, as in the Paleolithic diet. If you eat grains, you should choose the types which are the least processed: whole-wheat bread and cereal, sourdough bread, as well as whole-wheat or semi-whole-wheat rice and pasta.

Back to good health

For thousands of years, humans essentially consumed game (approximately 35% of the calorie intake) and wild plants such as leaves, roots, and berries (approximately 65% of the calorie intake). Anthony Sebastian, a professor of medicine at the University of California at San Francisco, evaluated the acid burden of this prehistoric diet, that is the net acid excretion (NAE), and compared it to that of our modern diet. We have gone from an average of 88 mEq per day– a very alkalizing diet – more than 10,000 years ago, to an average of +48 mEq per day – a clearly acidifying diet. We find ourselves in a context which is completely opposite to that of the first humans. However, genetically speaking, we do not differ from them: in order to function correctly, our body environment must be slightly alkaline. It is in our best interest to return to an alkalizing diet.

Cold cuts: zero to three portions weekly

You should not eat too many portions of cold cuts, as their high nitrate content increases the risk of colon cancer. Sausage, blood sausage, bologna, foie gras, pâtés, and hot dogs are moderately acidifying, whereas ham and salami are slightly more acidifying.

Fish and shellfish: three portions weekly

Like all animal protein, fish and shellfish are acidifying, but there are some differences between them. Fish and seafood that should be eaten in moderation include the following: canned salmon, salted cod, fish eggs, canned tuna in oil, carp, cuttlefish, fresh bluefin tuna (cooked), swordfish, canned sardines in oil, white tuna in oil, salmon, surimi, raw bluefin tuna, plain tuna, and pike. The least acidifying seafood include, in ascending order of acidification: oysters (especially when served with lemon!), grouper, pickled herring, wild salmon, lobster, turbot, scallops, octopus, fresh albacore tuna (cooked), whiting, cod, shrimps, mullet, rainbow trout, squid, and mackerel.

Dairy products: zero to two portions daily

The most acidifying dairy products are cheeses including parmesan, processed cheese, Swiss cheese, comté, gruyère, raclette, morbier, and goat's cheese. Less acidifying – and therefore a better choice if you like cheese – are the munster, cantal, mozzarella, roquefort, and saint-nectaire. Camembert, blue cheese, feta, reblochon, brie, and coulommiers are even less acidifying. Cottage cheese, yogurt, and milk are all moderately or slightly acidifying.

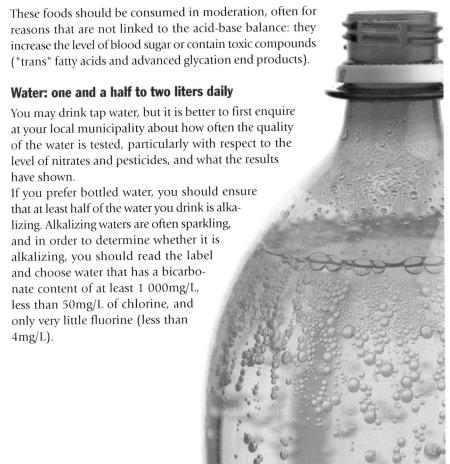

French fries, sweets, industrially-produced cake, pastries, sodas, salted and toasted nuts: zero to three portions weekly

These foods should be consumed in moderation, often for reasons that are not linked to the acid-base balance: they increase the level of blood sugar or contain toxic compounds ("trans" fatty acids and advanced glycation end products).

Water: one and a half to two liters daily

You may drink tap water, but it is better to first enquire at your local municipality about how often the quality of the water is tested, particularly with respect to the level of nitrates and pesticides, and what the results have shown.

If you prefer bottled water, you should ensure that at least half of the water you drink is alkalizing. Alkalizing waters are often sparkling, and in order to determine whether it is alkalizing, you should read the label and choose water that has a bicarbonate content of at least 1 000mg/L, less than 50mg/L of chlorine, and only very little fluorine (less than 4mg/L).

How can I reduce my consumption of salt?

A crucial element of a successful alkalizing diet is cutting down on salt. Everyone can reduce their salt consumption.

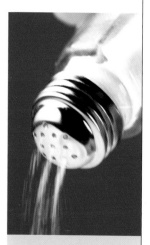

Where is salt hiding?

Salt occurring naturally in foods: 10%

Salt added during cooking or to dishes: 15%

Salt added during industrial production: 75%

It is not that simple to reduce your salt intake, as the saltshaker is not the real culprit. The cause of an excessive salt consumption is actually the salt "hidden" in industrially-produced foods, which represents between 70 and 80% of our total salt intake. As an excellent preservative and taste enhancer, it improves the taste and look of food. This is the reason why it is found everywhere, even where we least expect it: chocolate, biscuits, yogurt, dairy desserts, sodas, etc. The main carrier foods include bread, baked goods, cold cuts, soup, cheeses, ready-made meals, pizza, quiche, salty tarts, sandwiches, pastries, seafood, meat, poultry, condiments, and sauces. In order to reduce salt, use your common sense and consume fewer industrially-produced foods, which contain a lot of salt. Choose fresh products which you can cook at home, and go easy on the salt shaker.

How much sodium do you need?

Theoretically, you only need 2g of salt, that is 800mg of sodium daily to satisfy your body's needs. In the United States, health authorities recommend 2.4g of sodium (6g of salt) daily.

A few tips for reducing your salt intake

• Break the habit of always adding salt to your meals. In the beginning, food may seem bland, but with time, your taste buds will get accustomed to it. You will be able to discover the true taste of foods and you will take more pleasure in eating. You will also find that you start to spontaneously turn away from excessively salty foods. All you need to do is to follow your instinct. Replace salt with other condiments: garlic, parsley, celery, onion, thyme, herbs, and pepper. However, avoid mustard (it is very high in salt) and a host of other industrially-produced condiments, such as meat or chicken bouillon cubes, ready-made sauce bases, ketchup, and ready-made salad dressings. Use potassium-rich "salt".

Surprises in a can

	Potassium	Sodium
Raw green beans (100 g)	243 mg	4 mg
Cooked green beans (100 g)	240 mg	3 mg
Canned green beans (100 g)	107 mg	307 mg

Recommendations in the United States

In February 2004, the United States Institute of Medicine recommended an optimal consumption of approximately 1.5g of sodium and 2.3g of chloride daily, which results in a total of 3.8g of salt, of which we should not consume more than 5.8g daily.

• Limit your consumption of cold cuts, ready-made meals, canned foods, smoked fish, chips, crackers, and salted roast nuts and seeds.

• Rinse canned vegetables in order to get rid of most of the salt.

• Avoid adding salt to the water when you cook pasta, rice, or vegetables.

• Do not accustom your children to excessive amounts of salty food, as dietary habits begin forming during childhood and are difficult to change in adulthood.

Sources of sodium

Foods with a high salt content	Sodium
10 olives (30g)	600-900mg
1 portion of quiche Lorraine (130g)	680mg
1 slice of smoked ham (40g)	640mg
1 slice of Bayonne ham (40g)	560mg
30g of cereal, 1 chocolate croissant (80g)	350-400mg
1 portion of cooked milk cheese (30g)	330-350mg
1 portion of bleu cheese (15g)	240mg
1 slice of smoked salmon (20g)	240mg
1 slice of white bread (30g)	150mg
1 pint of milk	220mg

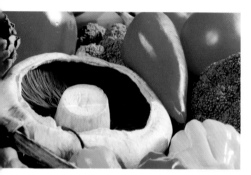

Potassium for your cells

Fruit and vegetables are our main source of potassium, and should be our first plan of action.

How much potassium do we need?

Contrary to vitamins, there is no recommended daily allowance for potassium. However, in February 2004, given the severity of health problems linked to the excessive consumption of industrially-produced foods and the insufficient consumption of fresh food, the United States Institute of Medicine recommended consuming "at least" 4.7g of potassium per day (see opposite table).

Recommended potassium intake

	Age	Men (g/day)	Women (g/day)
Babies	0 to 6 months	0,4	0,4
	7 to 12 months	0,7	0,7
Children	1 to 3 years	3,0	3,0
	4 to 8 years	3,8	3,8
	9 to 13 years	4,5	4,5
Adolescents	14 to 18 years	4,7	4,7
Adults	19 years and older	4,7	4,7
Pregnant women	14 to 50 years	-	4,7
Breastfeeding women	14 to 50 years	-	5,1

Where is potassium found?

There are many dietary sources of potassium, as it is the main building block of plant and animal cells (see table). Although meat, dairy products, and grains contain potassium, these foods generally acidify the body. It is therefore better to increase your consumption of plant products.

• Eat as many fruit and vegetables as you wish. Three to five servings of fruit and four to six servings of vegetables is ideal. The best sources of potassium (for 100kcal) are leafy green vegetables (spinach and lettuce), tomato, cucumber, zucchini, eggplant, winter squash, and root vegetables (carrots, radish, and turnips).

• Rediscover almonds, hazelnuts, and other nuts. As these foods contain a lot of fiber, they are rich in good fatty acids (unsaturated fatty acids) and are therefore an excellent source of potassium.

• As a snack, choose fruit, or if you must, fruit juice, although they contain less potassium. Choose ripe fruits, juice them and drink the fruit juice as soon as possible. In shops, choose 100% pure fruit juice with no added sugar.

Potassium content (mg/100 g)

Fat	0	Fresh avocado	522
Sugar	0	Fresh spinach	529
Egg	128	Baked potato	536
White bread	132	Raw black radish	554
Milk	150	Fresh chervil	600
Raspberry, blackberry, peach	220	Dates	670
Kiwi, cherry, gooseberry, grapes	280	Nuts	690
Whole-wheat bread	350	Dried lentils	700
Artichoke	350	Roast peanuts	710
Beef	370	Almonds	800
Banana, apricot, coconut	380	Dries prunes	950
Pork	390	Dried banana	1 150
Chocolate	400	Dried white kidney beans	1 450
Fish	400	Dried apricots	1 520
Mushrooms	420	Cocoa powder	1 920
Turkey	490	Red chili peppers	2 000
Veal	500		

Potassium salt and capsules

If you find it difficult to consume seven servings of fruit and vegetables a day, there are potassium supplements available which can remedy your deficiency.

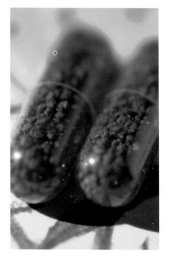

Swap table salt for potassium salt

Potassium salt is a dietetic salt which you can find at the pharmacy and use in the same way as your normal salt. It contains large amounts of potassium (30%), very little sodium (8%) and has the same taste as conventional salt. Note that in this type of salt, potassium is not bound to chloride but to bicarbonate, the form in which it is found in plant products (fruit and vegetables only contain small amounts of it)..

Potassium supplements

If your diet does not provide sufficient amounts of potassium, you can opt for supplements. Potassium capsules are available in pharmacies in the form of bicarbonate. If you are healthy, it is not dangerous to get more potassium from your diet than the recommended allowance, because excess potassium is simply excreted through the urine. The supplements are therefore not dangerous.

Who should not be taking potassium supplements?

People suffering from hyperkaliemia, or taking diuretics (the type which does not deplete the body of potassium), angiotensin-converting enzyme inhibitors, or digitalics should not take potassium supplements. In general, patients with impaired heart or kidney function, diabetics, and pregnant or breastfeeding women must consult their doctor before taking potassium supplements.

Monitor your magnesium levels

In order to remedy a potassium deficiency, your magnesium levels must be sufficient. Without magnesium, the cells cannot retain potassium.

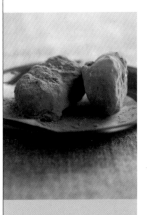

Magnesium is the second most important positive interstitial ion. Like potassium, it is found abundantly in all plant products. Magnesium is an alkalizing mineral which helps regain the acid-base balance.

Magnesium deficiency is a common problem

Magnesium is provided exclusively by our diet. However, our modern diet is far from covering our needs. According to a study carried out by the United States government, 68% of all Americans do not consume enough magnesium, and 19% do not even consume half of the recommended daily allowance. There are several reasons for this deficiency. Our modern diet contains a lot of processed foods and not enough plant products. Stress also generates physiological mechanisms which use up a lot of magnesium.

Dietary sources of magnesium

- Fruit and vegetables (almonds come in first with 275mg of magnesium per 100g).
- Chocolate: more than 300mg per 100g.
- Mineral water: Apollinaris, Pellegrino.

Magnesium supplements

You can buy magnesium carbonate capsules or dolomite capsules, which have the formula $CaMg(CO_3)_2$, in your pharmacy.

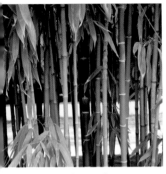

The alkalizing diet and osteoporosis

1. How it works

By re-establishing the body's acid-base balance, you reduce your excretion of calcium through the urine, slowing down bone degradation, thereby actively preventing osteoporosis and femoral head fractures.

2. My lifestyle recommendations

- Follow the alkalizing diet.
- To fight against osteoporosis, it is essential that the body gets enough calcium (1g/day). However, this is not sufficient. The absorption, retention, and binding of calcium in the bones depend on many parameters, such as the acid-base balance, vitamin D consumption, and physical activity.
- Consume less meat and cheese. Animal proteins acidify the blood, and force the body to re-establish your acid-base balance by depleting calcium reserves, or in other words, bone tissue.
- Be sure to consume enough vitamin D. Small quantities of this vitamin are found in food (cod liver oil, oily fish, and egg yolks). The body produces vitamin D through exposure to the sun (the skin produces it from cholesterol under the influence of ultraviolet rays). However, from October to April, supplements are essential, whether in the form of cod liver oil or vitamin D3 tablets.
- Remain active. People with sedentary lifestyles lose more calcium than those who exercise regularly. Exercise has an important role in bone growth. The traction on

Soy isoflavones

Numerous studies have shown that by taking an isoflavone supplement, women can slow down the loss of bone mass after menopause. One study has confirmed this observation by examining 177 women aged 49 to 65 years who were divided into two groups. The first group took 43mg of isoflavones for 1 year, while the second group took a placebo. Upon the study's completion, the women who had taken the isoflavones presented a higher bone mineral density in their lumbar vertebrae.

muscles and the consequent increased muscle mass stimulate bone growth. All sports are appropriate, with the exception of swimming, as it does not place enough stress on the bones.

3. My phyto-advice

Bamboo and **horsetail** are two plants that are very rich in silica. Silica is a mineral that allows calcium, phosphorous, and magnesium to bind to body tissues, as it promotes the absorption and binding of these minerals to bone tissue.

4. Pitfalls to avoid

Although dairy products are rich in calcium, one must avoid overconsumption. Cheese is generally very high in salt. Yogurt is therefore a better choice. Fortunately, there are many non-dairy sources of calcium, particularly leafy green vegetables. For example, 100g of Chinese cabbage contains more calcium than a glass of milk.

Sources of calcium in a healthy diet (mg/100g)

Plain yogurt	140-170	Green olives	100
Fresh sardines	290	Cooked spinach	256
Almonds	250	Chicory	100
Soy beans (mung beans)	255	Cooked broccoli	100
Fresh parsley	200	Egg yolk	140
Shrimp	200	Cooked white beans	60
Watercress	160	Cooked red beans	112
Nuts	175	**Beverages rich in calcium (mg/L)**	
Dried figs	160	Certain mineral waters	545

The alkalizing diet, rheumatism and gout

1. How it works

The acid crystals accumulated in the body act like grains of sand in the joints, and lead to joint degeneration. Joints lose their flexibility and become painfully inflamed.

2. My lifestyle recommendations

- Follow the alkalizing diet.
- Include anti-inflammatory spices in your cooking, such as ginger and turmeric. Ginger *(Zingiber officinale)* has been used for over 6,000 in India and China. Traditionally, it was used to treat digestive problems, as well as rheumatic pain. Traditional Indian medicine (Ayurvedic medicine) describes ginger as a reference plant to fight all types of inflammation. Very recent studies have confirmed the highly anti-inflammatory effects of the components in ginger. In fact, ginger appears to be as effective as modern anti-inflammatory drugs. Turmeric, or Indian saffron (*Curcuma longa*) is one of the main ingredients in curry, an essential mixture of spices in Indian cuisine. The Chinese name for turmeric literally means "yellow ginger", an allusion to the fact that it belongs to the same family as ginger. The roots of the turmeric plant are full of substances known as curcuminoids, including curcumin, which makes about 90% of the components in turmeric. Curcuminoids are known anti-oxidants and anti-inflammatory agents, which makes them extremely useful when recovering from surgery or fighting rheumatoid diseases.
- Consume anti-inflammatory fats, such as omega-3, which is found in oily fish, as well as in the form of fish oil capsules.
- Consume collagen, which slows cartilage degeneration. It can be found in chicken cartilage and shrimp shells.
- Remain active. Studies have shown that active individuals suffer less from joint pain, provided that they do not overwork their joints, of course! Choose physical activities that are not too hard on your joints, such as cycling or swimming.

3. My phyto-advice

Two plants should be included in your daily supplement routine: nettle and harpagophytum.

Harpagophytum (*Harpagophytum procumbens*) is harvested in the sandy deserts of South Africa and Namibia.

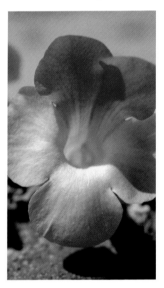

German botanists discovered the plant's analgesic and anti-inflammatory properties for the treatment of rheumatoid diseases in 1904. The dried root contains 0.5 to 3% of active substances, known as iridoids.

Nettle (*Urtica dioica*) was used by the Greeks and Romans, who used it to treat rheumatoid diseases. The leaves were consumed in the form of tea, soups, and salads. The German E Commi-ssion, which validates plant properties, recognizes the use of nettle leaves to treat inflammation and relieve rheumatic pain.

The alkalizing diet and fatigue

1. How it works

Chronic acidosis of the tissues and biological fluids places the body in a vicious cycle which causes the cells to remain in a state of energy deficiency. It slows down cells, creating a metabolic blockage. The body has barely enough energy to function.

2. My lifestyle recommendations

- Follow the alkalizing diet.
- Do not overeat. Eat until you are just about full. Eat in moderation every day, giving yourself permission to indulge from time to time.
- Make sure that you vary your diet! Do not eat the same things every day.
- Avoid becoming sedentary. Regular physical activity is the best way to ensure that you are in shape.

3. My phyto-advice

Plants rich in polyphenols are effective in fighting excess weight, as well as fatigue. I recommend two:
-Mate
-Green tea

Mate has not been well-known in North America for very long, but it is widely used in South America, where it is consumed regularly, just as Americans drink coffee. The medicinal properties of mate for fighting mental and physical fatigue are widely recognized. The theophylline and caffeine in mate leaves stimulate the heart muscle and central nervous system, relaxing the smooth muscles and improving peripheral blood circulation.

Tea is another well-known stimulant of the central nervous system. It contains caffeine and high levels of polyphenols. It also promotes mental activity and muscle performance.

4. Pitfalls to avoid

Ladies, watch your iron intake! One fourth of all American women of childbearing age suffer from iron deficiency, which will lead to chronic fatigue if not treated properly. To regain your energy, consume blood sausage, liver, and red meat.

Treatment against fatigue: Ginseng

Ginseng is a natural stimulant devoid of the negative effects of other stimulants such as caffeine and amphetamines. Ginseng has a tonifying and harmonizing effect, stimulating physical and mental energy. This is a plant that can be used if you feel tired after having worked too much, run around, or when you simply feel down. Ginseng allows you to maintain your energy levels during stressful and busy times. It is an excellent supplement to take when recovering from surgery or an energy-draining viral 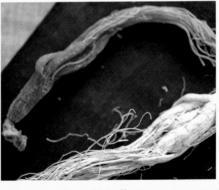 disease. Ginseng is recognized by the scientific community, and its effects are even more potent when it is taken in combination with vitamins.

The alkalizing diet and excess weight

1. How it works

Chronic acidosis promotes the development of abdominal fat and insulin resistance, which leads to a vicious cycle of weight gain.

2. My lifestyle recommendations

- Follow the alkalizing diet, increasing your protein intake, while decreasing sugars. By consuming proteins, you are forcing your body to spend much more energy than necessary for digesting fats or sugars. Moreover, proteins are filling. In order to lose weight, increase your protein intake so that it makes up 25% of your daily calorie intake, preferably eating vegetable proteins. The body will then use its fat reserves, while maintaining muscle mass.
- Exercise regularly. By increasing your muscle mass, you are using much more energy when at rest. Moreover, you are increasing fat-burning hormones such as testosterone and the growth hormone.

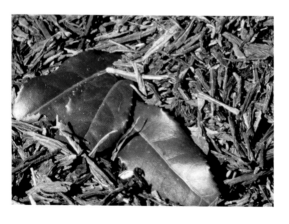

3. My phyto-advice

Four plants may be useful:
- Mate;
- *Citrus aurantium*;
- Green tea;
- Orthosiphon.

Mate leaves are rich in caffeine and saponin, which burn fat. Furthermore, mate slows down the progression of food through the stomach, making it an excellent appetite suppressant. Mate also has diuretic properties.

The rind of bitter orange (**Citrus aurantium**) contains synephrine, a substance which stimulates the receptors that "instruct" the body to burn fat in order to create energy. Three studies demonstrated that Citrus aurantium increases thermogenesis.

Green tea also increases energy expenditure by combining the action of caffeine and polyphenol (epigallocatechin gallate). Moreover, it stimulates the oxidation of fat.

Orthosiphon has powerful draining properties. Not only does it promote weight loss, but it also facilitates the elimination of toxins and waste, which would otherwise accumulate in the body and lead to fatigue and depression.

4. Pitfalls to avoid

- Avoid drastic low-calorie diets. These diets are very frustrating and cause you to lose more morale than pounds. These are often yo-yo diets: once you start eating normally again, your body will gain back the weight you lost.
- Do not eliminate too much fat from your diet. Studies have shown that over the long term (longer than 1 year), low-fat diets have no effect on body weight, as we need fats in our diet.

Do you feel like you need an appetite suppressant?

Fucus is a brown algae found on the rocky coasts of the cold and temperate seas of the Northern hemisphere. Because of its moist and sticky structure, the fucus thallus rehydrates in the stomach and expands in size, leading to a sensation of fullness. Fucus acts as a mechanical appetite suppressant, and also improves intestinal transit.

The alkalizing diet and type 2 diabetes

1. How it works

The alkalizing diet increases the intracellular pH, while decreasing fasting insulin levels. This decreases the risk of diabetes and diabetes complications. In addition, when we consume less salt and more potassium, we lower the amount of glucose absorbed by the intestines, improving the body's sensitivity to insulin, which has a positive effect on blood glucose regulation.

2. My lifestyle recommendations

- Follow the alkalizing diet on page 52.
- Eat several small meals per day in order to have more regular blood glucose levels. To slow down the absorption of blood glucose, you must:
• choose carbohydrates with a low glycemic index;
• reduce the total amount of sugars consumed,
• and increase fiber consumption.
- Every day, you should have two protein-rich meals:
• You should make sure you eat a healthy animal protein at lunch, for example, meat, poultry, or fish;
• Breakfast or dinner should include a different protein, possibly dairy or vegetables.

- Reduce your intake of saturated fat (fatty meat, sausages, and whole dairy products), and consume more high-quality vegetable oils, which are essential in avoiding complications from diabetes.
- Exercise every day (30 minutes per day is better than 2 hours only on Sunday!)

Dietary supplements

Omega-3: These fatty acids come from fish oil, and have proven effective in preventing cardiovascular disease. In addition, they increase cells' sensitivity to insulin, improving sugar metabolism.

Chromium: This trace element plays an important role in burning sugars. It stimulates insulin receptors, improving hormonal action.

Antioxidants: Zinc, selenium and vitamin E have shown positive effects on blood sugar and glycosylated hemoglobin levels over the long term.

3. My phyto-advice

Two plants have been proven effective against diabetes:
- olive blossom;
- fenugreek.

The **olive blossom** lowers blood sugar and increases diuresis. In addition, it decreases blood pressure, LDL (or "bad") cholesterol, triglycerides, and increases HDL ("good") cholesterol. Olive blossoms act not only against blood sugar, but are also beneficial for diabetics' fragile blood vessels. In addition, they have antioxidant properties.

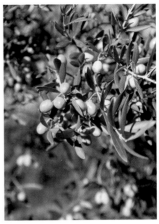

Fenugreek stimulates insulin secretion. A study conducted in 1990 by a team of French researchers effectively isolated the amino acid responsible for fenugreek's hypoglycemic effects.

4. Pitfalls to avoid

- Skipping meals
- Snacking between meals (if you cannot resist sweet treats, increase your physical activity).
- Many physicians recommend that their patients consume fructose instead of white sugar. The reason is that while both are sweeteners, fructose does not raise blood sugar. However, in animals, fructose leads to the occurrence of diabetes over the long term.
- Avoid artificial sweeteners, as sugar is sugar. Diabetics must make an enormous effort to get rid of their sweet tooth. They must not add sugar to drinks and food, even if they are artificial sweeteners, which are often high in sodium!

What is the glycemic index (GI)? *

The glycemic index is a reflection of a food's capacity to increase blood glucose levels. This value is indexed according to the identical quantity of a reference food, which is white bread. For example, when compared with white bread (GI 100), plain yogurt has a GI of 62, which is moderate, whereas a bar of chocolate has a GI of 80, which is rather high.

Glycemic Index for weight loss, Michel Montignac, Alpen Editions

The alkalizing diet and high blood pressure (HBP)

1. How it works

Chronic acidosis caused by a diet high in protein and low in potassium salts increases the stress hormone cortisol. Cortisol encourages the development of abdominal fat, which may make you vulnerable to insulin resistance. It leads to a series of problems, known as "syndrome X", which include obesity, diabetes or prediabetes, heart problems, high blood pressure, low levels of HDL or "good" cholesterol, and high triglycerides.

2. My lifestyle recommendations

- Follow the alkalizing diet on page 52.
- If you are overweight, it is essential that you lose weight. The alkalizing diet can help you with this.
- An excess consumption of alcohol is responsible for about 10% of HBP cases. Limit yourself to two glasses of red wine per day (one glass for women). Beyond that, alcohol is damaging to your health.
- Moderate but regular and prolonged physical exercise will allow you not only to control your weight, but also to reduce your blood pressure by 5 to 7mm. Endurance sports such as swimming, jogging, speedwalking, cross-country skiing, cycling, canoeing, and golf are recommended. Always consult your physician before starting any regular exercise program.

Potassium may prevent stroke

Epidemiological studies, such as a study from Harvard University, which was conducted on 43,000 Americans, suggest that people with high potassium levels (whether it is due to their diet alone or supplements) have a lower risk of stroke. Supplements may therefore also prevent stroke.

3. My phyto-advice

Three plants may be beneficial to you if you have moderately high blood pressure:
- the olive blossom;
- garlic;
- hawthorne.

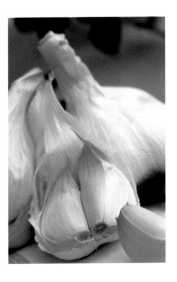

The leaf is the active part of the **olive blossom**. It is traditionally used by people in warm climates for its diuretic and hypotensive effects. The olive blossom also has antiarrhythmic and dilating effects on the coronary arteries. The olive blossom is particularly useful for moderate cases of high blood pressure, and as a curative or preventive treatment against a more severe form of high blood pressure with cardiovascular complications.

Garlic acts on blood platelets by decreasing their capacity to stick together. It thins the blood, improving circulation and preventing hypertension. Garlic is also an essential complement to the olive blossom.

Hawthorn is heart-friendly. This plant stimulates cardiac rhythm and, in a more general way, acts on the entire circulatory system. Hawthorne increases coronary blood flow and lowers blood pressure.

4. Pitfalls to avoid

- Stress tends to increase blood pressure. Therefore, either avoid stressful situations or learn to control your stress more effectively. Anyone can learn to manage their stress and relax!
- Regular consumption of licorice or products containing licorice can provoke or aggravate high blood pressure.

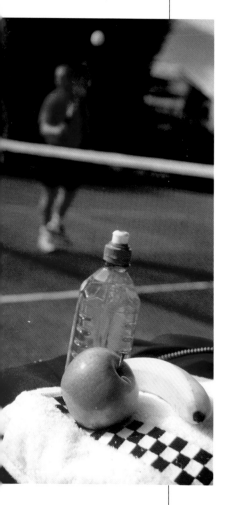

The alkalizing diet and muscle wasting

1. How it works

Acidosis leads to the degradation of muscle protein, which is not compensated for by increased protein synthesis. The urinary excretion of nitrogen, a component of protein, increases.

2. My lifestyle advice

- Follow the alkalizing diet on 52.
- Do not eat sugar or refined grains at night. These foods raise blood sugar, which lowers growth hormone levels. These hormones have an anabolic action which allows your body to retain or increase muscle mass.
- Take a potassium bicarbonate supplement (1 to 5g/day, according to your physician's recommendations). Potassium bicarbonate supplements decrease acidosis, which reduces the excretion of nitrogen through the urine. This spares muscle proteins from being broken down.
- Get regular exercise with one to three weight training sessions per week. Weight training stimulates growth hormone production.

3. My phyto-advice

Creatine is a natural substance which may be found in food (notably animal proteins).

Taken as a supplement, creatine facilitates short bursts of energy, which are needed in weight training. It allows you to lift heavy weights for a longer period of time, which results in increased muscle mass. Many studies have shown that creatine supplements improve muscle mass of athletes as well as that of sedentary and elderly people.

Potassium bicarbonate stimulates the growth hormone

The growth hormone is essential for the synthesis of muscle proteins. However, in developed countries, this hormone tends to decrease with age. According to one study, potassium bicarbonate supplements aimed at remedying chronic acidosis lead to a significant increase in growth hormone concentrations in the blood. Combined with regular exercise, this increase may be instrumental in conserving muscle mass in old age.

The alkalizing diet and asthma

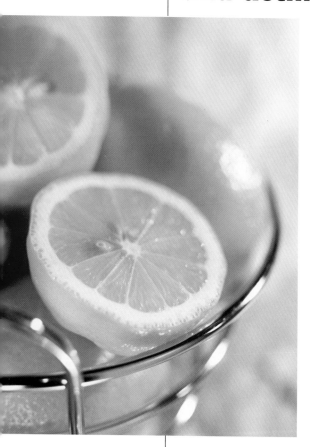

1. How it works

During an asthma attack, respiratory muscles must work very intensively. Under stress, they produce excessive amounts of lactic acid. In addition, as tissues lack oxygen and the volume of blood ejected by the heart is reduced, acidosis becomes even more pronounced. Therefore, it is essential that acidosis be treated.

2. My lifestyle recommendations:

- Follow the alkalizing diet on page 52.
- Eat large quantities of fruit and vegetables. Studies have shown that people who consume fruit and vegetables regularly suffer less from asthma and asthma attacks.
- Take potassium bicarbonate and magnesium supplements

regularly. These two factors remedy chronic acidosis. Many studies have found that asthmatics have a potassium deficiency, particularly during acute attacks. Therefore, researchers recommend taking potassium supplements.

3. My phyto-advice

According to numerous studies, vitamin C supplements may help fight against asthma attacks. In addition, the asthmatics' vitamin C reserves in the lungs tend to be depleted, and are therefore exposed to all kinds of oxidants.

GLOSSARY

Acid: A chemical substance which is capable of forming hydrogen ions by dissolving in water. Hydrochloric stomach acid, vinegar, and acetic acid are all examples of acids. An acid has a pH lower than 7.

Adenosine triphosphate (ATP): A substance made up of one molecule of adenine, one molecule of ribose, and three molecules of phosphate. ATP molecules are high in energy, and constitute the way in which energy produced by the combustion of sugars and fats is stored. This stored energy is released through the action of enzymes known as ATPases.

Amino acid: A component that makes up proteins. During digestion, proteins are broken down into amino acids. Twenty of them will be reused by the body to synthesize the proteins of our hair, skin, muscles, bones, blood, and other tissues and organs.

Anabolic: The property of a substance which facilitates muscle development. Insulin, the growth hormone, and testosterone are examples of anabolic hormones.

Base: A substance capable of neutralizing an acid by forming a salt. Sodium bicarbonate is an example of a base. Bases have a pH higher than 7.

Cortisol: A steroid hormone, secreted by the adrenal glands.

Enzyme: These are proteins which work on other substances in order to transform them. An enzyme is a biochemical tool which adds or takes away elements, modifies them, breaks down or forms molecules, etc. Like tools, enzymes need a key in order to be able to work. This key that activates them is known as a coenzyme. Many vitamins play the role of coenzymes, which explains the crucial role they have in the body. The substance that the enzyme works on is called a substrate. Enzymes may be recognized by their suffix "ase". For example, glucose oxidase is the enzyme responsible for oxidizing the glucose substrate; proteases break down proteins to "digest" them and allow them to be absorbed as amino acids; an elongase may elongate the carbon chain of fatty acids; a lysyl oxidase may link two collagen fibers, etc.

Hemoglobin: A pigment present in the red blood cells, necessary to transport oxygen from the lungs to the other parts of the body. Hemoglobin also returns carbonic acid stemming from energy production in the cells from sugars and fats.

Hormone: A chemical substance synthesized by endocrine glands (thymus, epiphysis, hypophysis, thyroid, parathyroid, adrenal glands, ovaries, testes, pancreas) or by certain tissues, which is released into the blood in order to be transported to the target organs, where it regulates different body functions.

Hypertension: Excessive increase in blood pressure. Blood pressure is expressed using two values. The first value, indicating systolic pressure, corresponds to the pressure of blood as it leaves the left ventricle and is pumped into the aorta. The second value is called diastolic pressure and indicates the pressure of blood that the arterial walls continue propulsing into peripheral areas while the heart is resting and filling up for the next contraction. A person is considered to suffer from hypertension when diastolic pressure is above 90mm of mercury (Hg). Your physician will provide these values in fractions: 14/9, 12/8, etc.

Lymph: Colorless liquid contained in the lymph vessels, which deposits waste from body tissues into venous blood.

Pral index (potential renal acid load): measured in milliequivalents (mEq), this index evaluates the acidity of urine – and therefore also the body's acidity – according to the quantity of acidic and alkaline minerals provided by our diet. As not all minerals are absorbed in the same way in the intestine, the Pral index has to take every mineral's intestinal absorption coefficient into account. This index adds acidic minerals and subtracts alkaline minerals. If you consume more acidifying than alkalizing minerals, the Pral index is higher than zero (positive) and your diet is acidifying. If it is the other way around, the Pral index is negative and your diet is alkalizing.

pH (potential of hydrogen): pH makes it possible to measure the hydrogen ion activity in a solution. This chemical scale measures the more or less acidic or alkaline property of a water-based solution. The lower the pH, the more acidic the solution is; the higher the pH, the more alkaline the solution is.

Purine: one of the azotic bases of nucleic acids (with pyrimidines), for example adenine and guanine.

Stroke: Cerebral neuronal damage caused by the obstruction of an artery or by hemorrhage.

BIBLIOGRAPHY

1 - D' LOWENSTEIN J., *Acid and Basics: a Guide to Understanding Acid-Base Disorders*, Jerome Lowenstein, New York, Oxford University Press, 1993.

2 - ROSE B.D., POST T.W., *Clinical Physiology of Acid-Base and Electrolyte Disorders*, Mc Graw-Hill International edition, 2001.

3 - REMER T., Influence of nutrition on acid-base balance – metabolic aspects, *Eur. J. Nutr.*, 2001 Oct, 40(5):214-220.

4 - FRASSETTO L., Diet, evolution and aging, *Eur. J. Nutr.*, 2001 Oct, 40(5):200-13.

5 - FRASSETTO L., MORRIS R.C. Jr et al., Diet, evolution and aging – the pathophysiologic effects of the post-agricultural inversion of the potassium-to-sodium and base-to-chloride ratios in the human diet, *Eur. J. Nutr.*, 2001 Oct, 40(5):200-13.

6 - MANN N.J., Paleolithic nutrition: what can we learn from the past? *Asia Pac. J. Clin. Nutr.*, 2004, 13(Suppl):S17.

7 - SEBASTIAN A., FRASSETTO L.A. et al., Estimation of the net acid load of the diet of ancestral preagricultural Homo sapiens and their hominid ancestors, *Am. J. Clin. Nutr.*, 2002 Dec, 76(6):1308-16.

8 - CORDAIN L., *The Paleo Diet*, John Wiley & Sons, 2003.

9 - BUSHINSKY D.A., Acid-base imbalance and the skeleton, *Eur. J. Nutr.*, 2001 Oct, 40(5):238-44.

10 - PRENTICE A., Diet, nutrition and the prevention of osteoporosis, *Public Health Nutr.*, 2004 Feb, 7(1A):227-43.

11 - BROWN S.E., JAFFE R., Acid-alkaline balance and its effect on bone health, *Int. J. of Integra Med.*, 2000, 2(6): 7-18.

12 - MACDONALD H.M., NEW S.A. et al., Low dietary potassium intakes and high dietary estimates of net endogenous acid production are associated with low bone mineral density in premenopausal women and increased markers of bone resorption in postmenopausal women, *Am. J. Clin. Nutr.*, 2005 Apr, 81(4):923-33.

13 - TUCKER K.L., HANNAN M.T., KIEL D.P., The acid-base hypothesis: diet and bone in the Framingham Osteoporosis Study, *Eur. J. Nutr.*, 2001 Oct, 40(5):231-7.

14 - REMER T., Manz F., High meat diet, acid-base status and calcium retention, *J. Nutr.*, 2003 Oct, 133(10):3239.

15 - FERRARI P., BONNY O., Diagnosis and prevention of uric acid stones, *Ther. Umsch.*, 2004, 61:571–574.

16 - GRASES F., Renal lithiasis and nutrition, *Nutr. J.*, 2006, 5:23.

17 - WANG S.Y., Related factors for hypokalemia during acute episode of bronchial asthma: clinical analysis in 56 children, *Di Yi Jun Yi Da Xue Xue Bao*, 2003, 23(8):867-869.

18 - CASO G., GARLICK P.J., Protein and amino acid metabolism, *Current Opinion in Clinical Nutrition & Metabolic Care*, January 2005, 8(1):73-76.

19 - Food and Nutrition Board, Institute of Medicine, *Potassium. Dietary Reference Intakes for Water, Potassium, Sodium, Chloride and Sulfate*, National Academies Press, Washington, D.C., 2004, 173-246.

20 - ATKINSON C., The effects of phytoestrogen isoflavones on bone density in women: a double-blind, randomised, placebo-controlled trial, *Am. J. Clin. Nutr.*, 2004, 79(2):326-333.

21 - *Prévention nutritionelle de l'ostéoporose* de Véronique Coxam & Marie Noêlle Horcapida. Page 69/71. Edition Lavoisier.

22 - Finer N : Energy Metabolism and Obesity. In : Salisbury J, dir., *Molecular Pathology*, Taylor & Francis, 2007. p. 23.

23 - McCARTY M.F., Acid-base balance may influence risk for insulin resistance syndrome by modulating cortisol output, *Med. Hypotheses*, 2005, 64 (2):380-4.

24 - FRASSETTO L., MORRIS R.C. Jr, SEBASTIAN A., Potassium bicarbonate increases serum growth hormone concentrations in postmenopausal women, *J. Am. Soc. Nephrol.*, 1996, 10:1349.

NOTES

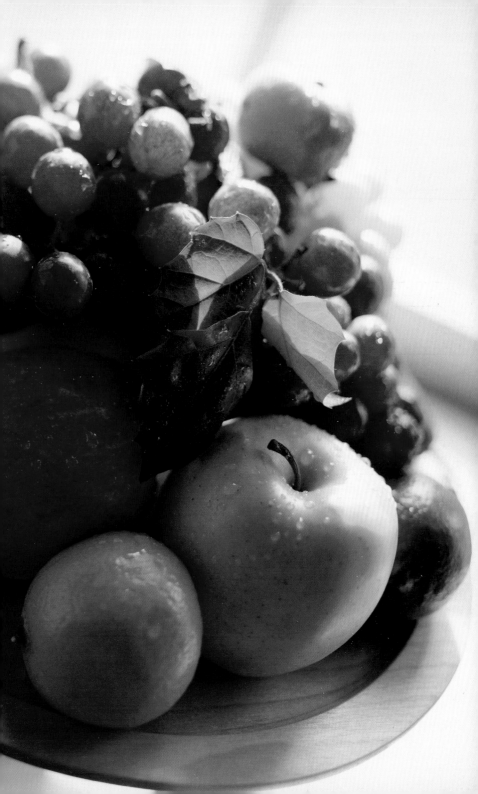

In our collection Alpen éditions:
-Osteoarthrisis, Rheumatism, Arthritis
-Osteoporosis
-Control your acidity, the acid/base diet
-Handle your menopause
-The Omega-3 Answer
-Living with a Hyperactive Child
-All About the Prostate
-The French Paradox
-The XXL Syndrome

with Michel Montignac:
-The French GI Diet for Women
-Eat Yourself Slim
-The Montignac Diet Cookbook
-The French GI Diet
-Glycemic Index Diet

www.alpen.mc